Keto Bread Machine Cookbook

300 Appetizing Bread Based Recipes for Ketogenic Goals. 21 Days Meal Plan Included

Table of Contents

Introduction

Baking bread is such an elemental process, I can't help but feel it is a deep, meditative connection to ages gone by. Combining wheat—the very essence of the earth—with water, salt from the sea, yeast from the air, and fire creates an alchemy that transforms the individual parts into much more than the whole. After baking so many loaves of bread, I now understand why all those scriptures, poems, stories, and fables make so much of bread and its importance to civilization and humanity. The truth of bread is that it requires a community and deep roots to exist. The farmer, the miller, the baker, and society itself, all working together toward a common goal. It is a beautiful ode to humankind and our ability to create magic with our own hands.

Baking is easier, and the results are best, when you have the proper tools and ingredients. In a perfect world, we'd all have kitchens equipped with every tool and gourmet ingredient that our heart desires. In the real world, most of us have space and budget limitations to consider. In this chapter I'll share which tools and ingredients I've found essential for baking, which ones are easy and inexpensive add-ons, and which fun stuff you might want to put on your "wish list."

Chapter 1. Basic Breads

1. Zucchini Baguettes

Servings: 2 big baguettes

Preparation Time: 30 Minutes

Calories: 481

Fat: 35.4 g

Protein: 24.9 g

Carbs: 9 g

Fiber: 1.2 g

Ingredients

5 eggs

3/4 cup zucchini, finely chopped

3/4 cup almond flour

2 tbsp. whole psyllium husks

1/2 cup sesame seeds

1/2 tsp. salt

1 1/2 tsp. baking powder

Direction

Preheat the oven to 375 F and line a baking sheet with parchment paper.

In a bowl, beat eggs with an electric mixer for about 3 minutes. Then add the grated zucchini and fold in thoroughly.

In another bowl, mix the dry ingredients, and blend thoroughly into the batter. Allow to rest for 10 minutes.

Shape 2 big baguettes with wet hands and place on the prepared baking sheet

Make 3 decorative cuts across the baguettes.

Bake in the middle of the oven for 30 minutes.

Cool and serve. Enjoy!

2. Mediterranean Baguettes

Servings: 2 big baguettes
Preparation Time: 30 Minutes
Calories: 488
Fat: 28.7 g
Protein: 25.8 g
Carbs: 7.4 g
Fiber: 2.2 g
Ingredients
5 eggs
100 g feta cheese, mashed
3/4 cup almond flour
2 tbsp. whole psyllium husks
2 tbsp. coconut flour
2 tbsp. dried Mediterranean oregano
1 tbsp. dried thyme
1 1/2 tsp. baking powder
Direction
Preheat the oven to 375 F. Line a baking sheet with parchment paper.

In a bowl, beat eggs with a hand mixer. Then fold mashed feta cheese into the batter.

In another bowl, mix dry ingredients, then blend thoroughly into the batter. Allow to rest for 10 minutes.

Shape 2 big baguettes with wet hands and place on the parchment-lined baking sheet.

Bake in the middle of the oven until golden brown, about 30 minutes.

Cool and serve. Enjoy!

3. Best Keto Bread

Servings: 20 Slices

Preparation Time: 30 Minutes

Calories: 90

Fat: 7 g

Protein: 3 g

Carbs: 2 g

Fiber: 1.5 g

Ingredients

1 1/2 cups almond flour

6 eggs, separated

4 tbsp. butter, melted

3 tsp. baking powder

1/4 tsp. cream of tartar

1 pinch pink salt

6 drops stevia

Direction

Preheat the oven to 375 F.

To the egg whites, add the cream of tartar and beat until soft peaks form.

In a food processor, add the salt, baking powder, almond flour, melted butter, and 1/3 of the beaten egg whites.

Mix until combined.

Add the remaining egg whites and process to mix. Don't over mix.

Pour in prepared (8 x 4loaf pan.

Bake for 30 minutes. Serve and enjoy!

4. Microwave Keto Bread

Servings: 1

Preparation Time: 5 Minutes

Calories: 220

Fat: 21 g

Protein: 4 g

Carbs: 4 g

Fiber: 1.7 g

Ingredients

3 tbsp. almond flour

1 egg

1 tbsp. butter

1/2 tsp. baking powder

Direction

Melt butter in the microwave in a bowl.

Add the egg, baking powder and almond flour to the butter Beat to mix well.

Microwave for 90 seconds.

Release from the bowl.

Slice in half and toast in the toaster. Serve and enjoy!

5. Almond Bread

Servings: 20

Preparation Time: 30 Minutes

Calories: 271

Fat: 22 g

Protein: 5 g

Carbs: 8 g

Fiber: 2.1 g

Ingredients

6 eggs, whites and yolk separated

1/4 tsp. cream of tatar

4 tbsp. butter, melted

3 tsp. baking powder

1 1/2 cups almond flour

Pinch salt

Direction

Preheat the oven to 375F.

Grease an 8 x 4-inch loaf pan and set aside.

In a bowl, beat egg whites and cream of tartar until soft peak starts to form.

Keep the mix on the side.

Add butter, egg yolks, baking powder, almond flour, and salt in a food processor and beat until mixed.

Add 1/3 of egg whites to the food processor and pulse until combined.

Add the rest in two steps and mix until well combined.

Transfer dough to the prepared loaf pan and bake for 30 minutes.

Cool and slice. Serve and enjoy!

6. Cinnamon Bread

Servings: 10
Preparation Time: 30 Minutes
Calories: 468
Fat: 45 g
Protein: 11 g
Carbs: 9 g
Fiber: 2.1 g
Ingredients
3 eggs
1 tsp. vinegar
3 tbsp. salted butter
2 tbsp. water
1/2 cup coconut flour
1/2 tsp. baking soda
1 tsp. cinnamon
1/2 tsp. baking powder
1/3 cup sour cream
1/8 tsp. stevia
Direction
Preheat the oven to 350F.
Grease a loaf pan and line the bottom with parchment paper.
Mix dry ingredients in a bowl and whisk well.
Add remaining ingredients to the dry mix and mix well.
Taste for sweetness. Adjust seasoning.
Let the mix stand for 3 minutes.
Spread batter into loaf pan and bake for 25 to 30 minutes.
Cool and load. Serve and enjoy!

7. Coconut Bread

Servings: 4

Preparation Time: 40 Minutes

Calories: 297

Fat: 14 g

Protein: 15 g

Carbs: 4 g

Fiber: 1.6 g

Ingredients

1 1/2 cups coconut flour

1/4 tsp. baking powder

1/8 tsp. salt

1 tbsp. coconut oil, melted

1 egg

Direction

Preheat the oven to 350F.

Add the coconut flour, baking powder, and salt to a bowl.

Add the oil, and eggs. Stir to mix.

Let the batter sit for several minutes.

Pour half the batter into the baking pan.

Spread it to form a circle, then repeat with remaining batter.

Bake in the oven for 10 minutes.

Once the bread has reached a golden brown texture, let it cool and serve. Enjoy!

8. Sandwich Bread

Servings: 8

Preparation Time: 45 Minutes

Calories: 146

Fat: 11 g

Protein: 5 g

Carbs: 7 g

Fiber: 1.2 g

Ingredients

1/2 cup sifted coconut flour

1/4 cup almond flour, sifted

6 eggs, whites and yolks separated

1/2 cup coconut oil

1/4 tsp. salt

3 tbsp. water

1 tbsp. apple cider vinegar

Direction

Preheat the oven to 350F.

Grease a (8 ½ by 4-inchloaf pan with oil.

Place a piece of parchment paper on the bottom of the pan.

Cream coconut oil in a food processor and add egg yolks at a time.

Pulse to combine coconut oil and yolks.

Add sifted coconut and almond flour, baking powder, apple cider vinegar, salt, and water to a food processor and pulse until combined.

Take a mixing bowl and beat egg whites.

Fold in coconut flour. Mix into egg whites and mix.

Pour the batter into prepared loaf pan and bake for 40 to 45 minutes.

Cover it with aluminum foil, about halfway through

Let it cool and then slice. Serve and enjoy!

9. Almond Bread 2

Servings: 8
Preparation Time: 60 Minutes
Calories: 277
Fat: 21 g
Protein: 10 g
Carbs: 7 g
Fiber: 0.8 g
Ingredients
3 cups almond flour
1 tsp. baking soda
2 tsp. baking powder
1/4 tsp. salt
1/4 cup almond milk
1/2 cup plus 2 tbsp. olive oil
3 eggs
Direction
Preheat the oven to 300F.
Grease a 9x5 inch loaf pan and put it to the side.
Add the listed ingredients in a bowl and mix well.
Transfer the batter to the prepared loaf pan.
Bake for 1 hour.
Remove and cool. Slice serve and enjoy!

10. Multi-Purpose Keto Bread

Servings: 12
Preparation Time: 1 Hour 30 Minutes
Calories: 350
Fat: 21 g
Protein: 17 g
Carbs: 9 g
Fiber: 1.8 g
Ingredients
6 egg whites
2 eggs whole
1/2 cup coconut flour
1 1/2 cups sesame seed flour
1/3 cup psyllium husk powder
1 tbsp. baking powder
1/2 to 1 tsp. salt
2 cups boiling water
Direction
Preheat the oven to 350F.
Line a loaf pan with parchment paper and set aside.
Whisk egg whites and whole eggs.
Combine dry ingredients, and egg mix.
Place in a mixer, and combine to make a thick dough.
Gradually pour in boiling water and mix well.
Transfer mix to prepared loaf pan and bake for 90 minutes.
Remove and cool. Serve and enjoy!

11. Eggy Coconut Bread

Servings: 4

Preparation Time: 40 Minutes

Calories: 297

Fat: 14 g

Protein: 15 g

Carbs: 9 g

Fiber: 3.1 g

Ingredients

4 eggs

1 cup water

2 tbsp. apple cider vinegar

1/4 cup plus 1 tsp. coconut oil, melted

1/2 tsp. garlic powder

1/2 cup coconut flour

1/2 tsp. baking soda

1/4 tsp. salt

Direction

Preheat the oven to 350F.

Grease a baking tin with 1 tsp. coconut oil. Set aside.

Add eggs to a blender along with vinegar, water, and ¼-cup coconut oil. Blend for 30 seconds.

Add coconut flour, baking soda, garlic powder, and salt. Blend for 1 minute.

Transfer to the baking tin.

Bake for 40 minutes. Serve and enjoy!

12. Coconut Flatbread

Servings: 4

Preparation Time: 10 Minutes

Calories: 297

Fat: 14 g

Protein: 15 g

Carbs: 5 g

Fiber: 2.9 g

Ingredients

1 1/2 tbsp. coconut flour

1/4 tsp. baking powder

1/8 tsp. salt

1 tbsp. coconut oil, melted

1 egg

Direction

Preheat the oven to 350F.

In a bowl, add coconut flour, baking powder, and salt.

Add eggs and coconut oil and stir well to mix.

Let the batter sit for several minutes.

Pour half the batter into the baking pan.

Spread it to form a circle, then repeat with the remaining batter.

Bake in the oven for 10 minutes.

Once baked, remove and cool. Serve and enjoy!

13. Keto Garlic Bread

Servings: 20

Preparation Time: 20 Minutes

Calories: 230

Fat: 27 g

Protein: 8 g

Carbs: 1 g

Fiber: 1.2 g

Ingredients

1 1/4 cups almond flour

5 tbsp. psyllium husk powder

2 tsp. baking powder

1 tsp. salt

2 tsp. apple cider vinegar

1 cup boiling water

3 egg whites

4 oz. butter

1 garlic clove

2 tbsp. chopped parsley

1/2 tsp. salt

Direction

Preheat your oven at 375 degrees Fahrenheit.

Mix the almond flour, psyllium husk powder, baking powder and the salt.

Boil the water and mix it with the apple cider vinegar and the egg whites.

Mix the dry ingredients to the wet ingredients and form the dough.

Make 10 buns with the dough and place them on a greased baking sheet.

Put the buns to bake in preheated oven for 40 to 50 minutes or until they turn golden brown.

Make the garlic butter by mixing the melted butter, crushed garlic, chopped parsley and the salt.

Brush this mixture on the buns and serve. Enjoy!

14. Keto BLT With Oopsie Bread

Servings: 20

Preparation Time: 20 Minutes

Calories: 230

Fat: 30 g

Protein: 5 g

Carbs: 0.5 g

Fiber: 1 g

Ingredients

3 eggs

4 1/2 oz. cream cheese

Pinch salt

1/2 tbsp. psyllium husk powder

1/2 tsp. baking powder

8 tbsp. mayonnaise

5 oz. bacon

2 oz. lettuce

1 tomato, sliced

Few basil

Direction

Preheat your oven at 300 degrees Fahrenheit.

Separate the egg yolks and the egg whites.

Beat the egg whites with the salt until the soft foaming mixture emerges.

Mix the cream cheese with the egg yolks.

Now mix in the baking powder and the psyllium husk powder.

Now fold the egg whites in the egg yolk mixture.

Put the oopsies on a greased baking tray.

Put it to bake in preheated oven for 25 minutes or until they turn golden brown.

For the BLT, fry the bacon pieces until they turn crispy.

Spread the mayonnaise on the oopsie bread.

Now place over the lettuce, sliced tomatoes and chopped basil on top.

Finally, put over the fried bacon pieces. Serve and enjoy!

15. Oopsie Bread Rolls

Servings: 6

Preparation Time: 20 Minutes

Calories: 255

Fat: 27 g

Protein: 10 g

Carbs: 0.9 g

Fiber: 1 g

Ingredients

3 eggs

1/8 tsp. cream of tartar

3 oz. cream cheese

1/8 tsp. salt

Direction

Preheat your oven at 300 degrees Fahrenheit.

Separate the egg yolks and the egg whites.

Whip the egg whites with the cream of tartar until soft peaks form.

Now in another bowl mix the egg yolks, cream cheese and the salt.

Now fold the egg whites in to the egg yolk mixture.

Pour the batter on to a greased pan and put to bake in preheated oven for 30 minutes.

Cool for a few minutes and then serve. Enjoy!

16. Healthy Cornbread

Servings: 6

Preparation Time: 20 Minutes

Calories: 152

Fat: 21 g

Protein: 7 g

Carbs: 1.8 g

Fiber: 2.3 g

Ingredients

1 cup coconut flour

1 tsp. swerve

1 tsp. Celtic sea salt

3 1/2 tsp. baking powder

5 eggs

1/2 cup vanilla almond milk

1/3 cup coconut oil

1 can baby corn

Direction

Preheat your oven at 350 degrees Fahrenheit.

Mix together the coconut flour, salt and the baking powder.

Now add in the swerve, eggs, vanilla almond milk and the coconut oil.

Fold in the baby corns.

Pour the batter in to a prepared pan and put to bake in preheated oven for 30 to 35 minutes or until it turns golden brown.

Cool and serve. Enjoy!

17. Coconut And Almond Bread

Servings: 12

Preparation Time: 10 Minutes

Calories: 192

Fat: 31 g

Protein: 9 g

Carbs: 1.1 g

Fiber: 2 g

Ingredients

1 1/2 cups almond flour

2 tbsp. coconut flour

1/4 cup flaxseeds

1/4 tsp. salt

1 1/2 tsp. baking soda

5 eggs

1/4 cup coconut oil

1 tsp. sweetener

1 tbsp. apple cider vinegar

Direction

Preheat your oven at 350 degrees Fahrenheit.

Mix together the dry ingredients; almond flour, coconut flour, flax seeds, sweetener, salt and the baking soda.

Now add in the eggs, coconut oil and the apple cider vinegar. Pour the batter in to a greased loaf pan and then put to bake in preheated oven for 30 minutes or until done.

Cool it and then serve. Enjoy!

18. Focaccia Style Flax Bread

Servings: 12

Preparation Time: 15 Minutes

Calories: 222

Fat: 30 g

Protein: 8 g

Carbs: 0.8 g

Fiber: 2 g

Ingredients

2 cups flax seed meal

1 tbsp. baking powder

1 tsp. salt

2 tbsp. sugar

5 eggs

1/2 cup water

1/3 cup oil

Direction

Preheat your oven at 350 degrees Fahrenheit.

Mix together the flax seed meal, baking powder, salt and sugar.

Now add the eggs, water and oil and mix well.

Leave the batter for a few minutes to thicken up and then pour it in to a prepared greased pan.

Put the pan to bake in preheated oven for 30 minutes or until when it is browned.

Cool and then cut. Enjoy!

19. Low Carb Bun For One

Servings: 1

Preparation Time: 10 Minutes

Calories: 232

Fat: 27 g

Protein: 9 g

Carbs: 0.3 g

Fiber: 2 g

Ingredients

1 tbsp. coconut oil

1 egg

1 tbsp. coconut milk

1 tbsp. almond flour

1 tbsp. coconut flour

1/8 tsp. baking soda

Sesame seeds, for sprinkling over

Direction

Blend together the coconut oil, egg, coconut milk, almond flour, coconut flour and the baking soda.

Mix everything well and then pour the batter in to a greased cake pan.

Preheat your oven at 350 degrees Fahrenheit.

Put the cake pan in preheated oven for about 18 to 20 minutes.

If you want to prepare the bun in microwave, you can make it in 2 minutes or even less.

Sprinkle over the sesame seeds on top.

Cool and then serve. Enjoy!

20. 5 Ingredient Chocolate Chip Keto Bread

Servings: 2

Preparation Time: 8 Minutes

Calories: 222

Fat: 36 g

Protein: 11 g

Carbs: 4.5 g

Fiber: 1.7 g

Ingredients

2 scoops protein powder

2 eggs, separated

2 tbsp. butter

Pinch salt

50 g cocao nibs

1/2 cup maple syrup

Direction

Beat the egg whites until stiff peaks form.

In another bowl, mix the egg yolks, protein powder and the butter.

Now fold in the egg whites in to this mixture.

Now add in the salt and the cacao nibs. Mix well.

Preheat your oven at 350 degrees Fahrenheit.

Pour this mixture in to a greased cake pan and bake until it turns golden brown for approximately 25 minutes.

Serve warm and drizzle over maple syrup. Enjoy!

21. Peanut Butter And Chocolate Bread

Servings: 6

Preparation Time: 20 Minutes

Calories: 187

Fat: 46 g

Protein: 7.9 g

Carbs: 3.1 g

Fiber: 2 g

Ingredients

1 cup almond flour

1/2 cup erythritol

1 tsp. baking powder

Pinch salt

1/3 cup peanut butter

1/3 cup almond milk

2 eggs

1/2 cup cacao nibs

Direction

Mix together the almond flour, erythritol, baking powder and the salt.

Now add in the peanut butter, almond milk and the eggs.

Mix well. Lastly fold in the cacao nibs and put the mixture in to a prepared greased pan.

Preheat your oven at 350 degrees Fahrenheit and put the pan to bake in the preheated oven for 25 minutes or until the cake is cooked. Serve and enjoy!

22. Low Carb Vanilla Bread

Servings: 5

Preparation Time: 10 Minutes

Calories: 198

Fat: 33 g

Protein: 6.8 g

Carbs: 2.3 g

Fiber: 2 g

Ingredients

5 eggs, separated

4 tbsp. coconut flour

4 tbsp. granulated sweetener

1 tsp. baking powder

2 tsp. vanilla extract

3 tbsp. full fat milk

125 g melted butter

Direction

Separate the egg whites and the egg yolks and beat the egg whites until they form in to stiff peaks.

In another bowl, beat the egg yolks, coconut flour, granulated sweetener and the baking powder.

Now slowly and gradually pour in the melted butter carefully and mix it to make sure that you have a very smooth consistency of your batter.

Next, add in the full fat milk and the vanilla extract.

With the help of a rubber spatula, now very gently fold in the egg whites in the mixture.

Try to keep as much as air and fluffiness that you can for better results.

Preheat your oven at 350 degrees Fahrenheit and put the pan to bake in preheated oven for 30 minutes or until it is golden brown,

Cool and then serve. Enjoy!

23. Chocolate Bread

Servings: 1

Preparation Time: 5 Minutes

Calories: 258

Fat: 39 g

Protein: 12 g

Carbs: 4 g

Fiber: 2 g

Ingredients

2 tbsp. cocoa powder

1/2 cup almond flour

2 tbsp. erythritol

1 egg

1 tbsp. heavy cream

1/2 tsp. vanilla extract

1/4 tsp. baking powder

Pinch salt

Direction

Preheat your oven at 350 degrees Fahrenheit.

Whisk together the cocoa powder, almond flour and the sweetener erythritol and make sure to remove lumps.

In another bowl, beat the egg well.

Now add the egg, heavy cream and the vanilla extract in to the erythritol mixture and mix.

Add in the salt and baking powder as well.

Mix all the ingredients properly.

Grease your pan, pour the batter in and then put it to bake in preheated oven for 10 to 15 minutes or until the bread is done.

Serve bread when it cools down. Enjoy!

24. Whole Wheat Coconut Bread

Servings: 8

Preparation Time: 10 Minutes

Calories: 228

Fat: 34.5 g

Protein: 8.6 g

Carbs: 2.6 g

Fiber: 1.8 g

Ingredients

1 1/2 cups pastry flour

2 tbsp. sugar

2 tsp. baking powder

1/2 tsp. salt

1 1/2 cups milk

1/3 cup melted coconut oil

1 egg

1/2 tsp. vanilla extract

Direction

Preheat your oven at 350 degrees Fahrenheit.

Mix together the pastry flour, sugar, baking powder and salt.

Make a well in the center and add in the wet ingredients that are milk, melted coconut oil, egg and vanilla extract.

Pour the batter in to a greased cake pan and cook until the bread turns golden brown for approximately 25 minutes.

Cool and serve. Enjoy!

25. Keto Blueberry Lemon Bread

Servings: 16

Preparation Time: 30 Minutes

Calories: 308

Fat: 35 g

Protein: 6 g

Carbs: 1.6 g

Fiber: 1.8 g

Ingredients

3 cups almond flour

2 tbsp. egg white protein powder

1 tsp. cream of tartar

1/2 tsp. baking soda

1/4 tsp. Celtic sea salt

6 eggs

1 tbsp. lemon zest

1/2 tbsp. vanilla extract

1/2 tsp. vanilla stevia

1 cup blueberries

Direction

In a food processor, blend together the almond flour, egg white protein powder, cream of tartar, baking soda and the salt.

Now add in the eggs, lemon zest, vanilla extract and the vanilla stevia.

Next, fold in the blue berries.

Mix the batter well and then pour the batter in to a prepared greased pan.

Preheat your oven at 350 degrees Fahrenheit.

Put the pan to bake in preheated oven for 45 to 50 minutes or until baked to perfection.

Cool and then serve. Enjoy!

26. Low Carb Baked Bread

Servings: 12
Preparation Time: 15 Minutes
Calories: 263
Fat: 25 g
Protein: 15 g
Carbs: 1.3 g
Fiber: 1.2 g
Ingredients
2 1/2 cups almond flour
2 tsp. baking powder
1/4 tsp. baking soda
1/4 tsp. salt
1/4 cup softened butter
2 tbsp. egg white protein powder
3 eggs
4 tsp. Anise extract
Direction
Preheat your oven at 350 degrees Fahrenheit.
Mix almond flour, baking powder, baking soda and salt in a bowl.
In a separate bowl, beat the butter.
Now add in the eggs, anise extract and beat them with butter.
Now mix in the flour and the egg white protein powder and form the dough.
Cut the dough lengthwise and place the slices on to a prepared baking sheet.
Put the slices to bake in preheated oven for about 10 minutes or until both sides turn brown.
Cool and serve. Enjoy!

27. Caprese On Toast

Servings: 14

Preparation Time: 15 Minutes

Calories: 280

Fat: 27 g

Protein: 11.3 g

Carbs: 2.3 g

Fiber: 0.4 g

Ingredients

14 slices sourdough bread

2 garlic cloves

1 pound mozzarella cheese

1/3 cup fresh basil leaves

3 tomatoes

3 tbsp. extra virgin olive oil

Pinch salt

Pinch pepper

Direction

Cut your sourdough bread in to 14 slices and toast them until both sides turn brown.

Rub garlic on both sides of the bread.

Top each with a slice of mozzarella cheese.

Now place a slice of tomato and basil leaves on each bread slice.

Drizzle olive oil and sprinkle salt and pepper on top. Serve and enjoy!

28. Blackberry Bread

Servings: 4

Preparation Time: 10 Minutes

Calories: 102

Fat: 19.8 g

Protein: 5.3 g

Carbs: 0.9 g

Fiber: 0.7 g

Ingredients

5 eggs

1 tbsp. butter

3 tbsp. coconut flour

1 tsp. grated ginger

1/4 tsp. vanilla

1/3 tsp. salt

1/2 orange zest

1 tsp. chopped rosemary

1/2 cup fresh blackberries

Direction

Preheat your oven at 350 degrees Fahrenheit.

Blend properly, the eggs, butter, coconut flour, grated ginger, vanilla, salt and the orange zest in a blender.

Then add in the rosemary and blend.

Pour the mixture in to a loaf pan and sprinkle over some blueberries.

Place the loaf pan for baking in a preheated oven for 25 minutes or until the bread achieves a perfect golden color.

Cut perfect slices and enjoy every bite of the soft blackberry bread once it cools down.

29. Garlic, Herb And Cheese Bread

Preparation time: 5 minutes

Servings: 12

Ingredients:

½ cup ghee

6 eggs

2 cups almond flour

1 tsp baking powder

½ tsp xanthan gum

1 cup cheddar cheese, shredded

1 tbsp garlic powder

1 tbsp parsley

½ tbsp. oregano

½ tsp salt

Directions:

Lightly beat eggs and ghee before pouring into bread machine pan.

Add the remaining ingredients to the pan.

Set bread machine to gluten free.

When the bread is done, remove bread machine pan from the bread machine.

Let cool slightly before transferring to a cooling rack.

You can store your bread for up to 5 days in the refrigerator.

Nutrition:

Calories 156

Carbohydrates 4 g

Fats 13 g

Sugar 4g

Protein 5 g

30. Pumpkin And Sunflower Seed Bread

Preparation time: 8 minutes
Servings: 10

Ingredients:
½ cup ground psyllium husk
½ cup chia seeds
½ cup pumpkin seeds
½ cup sunflower seeds
2 tbsp ground flaxseed
1 tsp baking soda
¼ tsp salt
3 tbsp coconut oil, melted
1 ¼ cup egg whites
½ cup almond milk
Directions:
Place all wet ingredients into bread machine pan first.
Add dry ingredients.
Set bread machine to the gluten free setting.
When the bread is done, remove bread machine pan from the bread machine.
Let cool slightly before transferring to a cooling rack.
You can store your bread for up to 5 days in the refrigerator.
Nutrition:
Calories 155
Carbohydrates 4 g
Fats 8 g
Sugar 3g
Protein 5 g

31. Rosemary Bread

Preparation time: 4 minutes
Servings: 12

Ingredients:
2 ½ cups almond flour
¼ cup coconut flour
½ cup ghee
8 oz cream cheese
5 eggs
1 tsp rosemary
1 tsp sage, ground
2 tsp parsley
1 tsp baking powder
Directions:
Slightly beat eggs and ghee together in a bowl then pour into bread machine pan.
Add all the remaining ingredients.
Set bread machine to the French bread setting
When the bread is done, remove bread machine pan from the bread machine.
Let cool slightly before transferring to a cooling rack.
You can store your bread for up to 7 days in the refrigerator.
Nutrition:
Calories 140
Carbohydrates 2.8 g
Fats 14 g
Protein 5 g

32. Savory Herb Blend Bread

Preparation time: 7 minutes
Servings: 16

Ingredients:
1 cup almond flour
½ cup coconut flour
1 cup parmesan cheese
¾ tsp baking powder
3 eggs
3 tbsp coconut oil
½ tbsp rosemary
½ tsp thyme, ground
½ tsp sage, ground
½ tsp oregano
½ tsp garlic powder
½ tsp onion powder
¼ tsp salt
Directions:
Light beat eggs and coconut oil together before adding to bread machine pan.
Add all the remaining ingredients to bread machine pan.
Set bread machine to the gluten free setting.
When the bread is done, remove bread machine pan from the bread machine.
Let cool slightly before transferring to a cooling rack.
You can store your bread for up to 7 days .
Nutrition:
Calories 170
Carbohydrates 6 g
Fats 15 g
Protein 9 g

33. Cinnamon Almond Bread

Preparation time: 3 minutes

Servings: 10

Ingredients:

2 tbsps. coconut flour

1 tsp baking soda

2 cups almond flour

2 tbsps. coconut oil

¼ cup flaxseed, ground

1 egg white

1 ½ tsp lemon juice

5 eggs

2 tbsps. erythritol

½ tsp salt

1 tbsp. cinnamon

Directions:

Pour wet ingredients into bread machine pan.

Add dry ingredients to the bread machine pan.

Set bread machine to the gluten free setting.

When the bread is done, remove bread machine pan from the bread machine.

Let cool slightly before transferring to a cooling rack.

You can store your bread for up to 5 days.

Nutrition:

Calories 220

Carbohydrates 10 g

Fats 15 g

Protein 9 g

34. Cheesy Garlic Bread

Preparation time: 30 minutes
Servings: 10

Ingredients:
¾ cup mozzarella, shredded
½ cup almond flour
2 tbsps. cream cheese
1 tbsp. garlic, crushed
1 tbsp. parsley
1 tsp baking powder
Salt, to taste
1 egg
For the toppings:
2 tbsps. melted butter
½ tsp parsley
1 tsp garlic clove, minced
Directions:
Mix together your topping ingredients and set aside.
Pour the remaining wet ingredients into the bread machine pan.
Add the dry ingredients.
Set bread machine to the gluten free setting.
When the bread is done, remove bread machine pan from the bread machine.
Let cool slightly before transferring to a cooling rack.
Once on a cooling rack, drizzle with the topping mix.
You can store your bread for up to 7 days.
Nutrition:
Calories: 29
Carbohydrates: 1g
Protein: 2g
Fiber 1g
Fat: 2g

35. Almond Flour Bread

Preparation time: 4 minutes
Servings: 10

Ingredients:
4 egg whites
2 egg yolks
2 cups almond flour
¼ cup butter, melted
2 tbsp psyllium husk powder
1 ½ tsp baking powder
½ tsp xanthan gum
Salt
½ cup + 2 tbsps. warm water
2 ¼ tsp yeast
Directions:
Use a small mixing bowl to combine all dry ingredients, except for the yeast.
In the bread machine pan add all wet ingredients.
Add all of your dry ingredients, from the small mixing bowl, in the bread machine pan. Top with the yeast.
Set the bread machine to the basic bread setting.
When the bread is done, remove bread machine pan from the bread machine.
Let cool slightly before transferring to a cooling rack.
The bread can be stored for up to 4 days on the counter and for up to 3 months in the freezer.
Nutrition:
Calories 110
Carbohydrates 2.4 g
Fats 10 g
Protein 4 g

36. Coconut Flour Bread

Preparation time: 5 minutes
Servings: 12

Ingredients:

6 eggs

½ cup coconut flour

2 tbsp psyllium husk

¼ cup olive oil

1 ½ tsp salt

1 tsp xanthan gum

1 teaspon baking powder

2 ¼ tsp yeast

Directions:

Use a small mixing bowl to combine all dry ingredients, except for the yeast.

In the bread machine pan add all wet ingredients.

Add all of your dry ingredients, from the small mixing bowl, in the bread machine pan. Top with the yeast.

Set the bread machine to the basic bread setting.

When the bread is done, remove bread machine pan from the bread machine.

Let cool slightly before transferring to a cooling rack.

The bread can be stored for up to 4 days on the counter and for up to 3 months in the freezer.

Nutrition:

Calories 174

Carbohydrates 4 g

Fats 15 g

Protein 7 g

37. Cloud Bread Loaf

Preparation time: 5 minutes
Servings: 10

Ingredients:
6 egg whites
6 egg yolks
½ cup whey protein powder, unflavored
½ tsp cream of tartar
6 oz sour cream
½ tsp baking powder
¼ tsp garlic powder
¼ tsp onion powder
¼ tsp salt
Directions:
Using a hand mixer beat egg whites and cream of tartar together until you have stiff peaks forming. Set aside.
Combine all other ingredients into another bowl and mix together.
Fold the mixtures together, a little at a time.
Pour mixture into your bread machine pan.
Set the bread machine to quick bread.
When the bread is done, remove bread machine pan from the bread machine.
Let cool slightly before transferring to a cooling rack.
The bread can be stored for up to 3 days on the counter.
Nutrition:
Calories 90
Carbohydrates 2 g
Fats 7 g
Protein 6 g

38. Sourdough Bread

Preparation time: 6 minutes
Servings: 10

Ingredients:
½ cup almond flour
½ cup coconut flour
½ cup ground flaxseed
1/3 cup psyllium husk powder
1 tsp baking soda
1 tsp Himalayan salt
2 eggs
6 egg whites
¾ cup buttermilk
¼ cup apple cider vinegar
½ cup warm water
Directions:
Combine the flours, flaxseed, psyllium husk, baking soda, and salt into a bowl, mix together, and set aside.
Place eggs, egg whites, and buttermilk into bread machine baking pan.
Add dry ingredients on top, then pour over vinegar and warm water.
Set bread machine to French setting (or a similar longer setting).
Check dough during kneading process to see if more water may be needed.
When the bread is done, remove bread machine pan from the bread machine.
Let cool slightly before transferring to a cooling rack.
The bread can be stored for up to 10 days in the fridge or for 3 months in the freezer.
Nutrition:
Calories 85
Carbohydrates 4 g
Fats 4 g
Protein 6 g

39. Seeded Loaf

Preparation time: 5 minutes
Servings: 16

Ingredients:
7 eggs
1 cup almond flour
½ cup butter
2 tbsp olive oil
2 tbsp chia seeds
2 tbsp sesame seeds
1 tsp baking soda
½ tsp xanthan gum
¼ tsp salt
Directions:
Add eggs and butter to the bread machine pan.
Top with all other ingredients.
Set bread machine to the gluten free setting.
Once done remove from bread machine and transfer to a cooling rack.
This bread can be stored in the fridge for up to 5 days or 3 weeks in the freezer.
Nutrition:
Calories 190
Carbohydrates 8 g
Fats 18 g
Protein 18 g

40. Simple Keto Bread

Preparation time: 3 minutes

Servings: 8

Ingredients:

3 cups almond flour

2 tbsp inulin

1 tbsp whole milk

½ tsp salt

2 tsp active yeast

1 ¼ cups warm water

1 tbsp olive oil

Directions:

Use a small mixing bowl to combine all dry ingredients, except for the yeast.

In the bread machine pan add all wet ingredients.

Add all of your dry ingredients, from the small mixing bowl, in the bread machine pan. Top with the yeast.

Set the bread machine to the basic bread setting.

When the bread is done, remove bread machine pan from the bread machine.

Let cool slightly before transferring to a cooling rack.

The bread can be stored for up to 5 days on the counter and for up to 3 months in the freezer.

Nutrition:

Calories 85

Carbohydrates 4 g

Fats 7 g

Protein 3 g

41. Classic Keto Bread

Preparation time: 3 minutes
Servings: 10

Ingredients:
7 eggs
½ cup ghee
2 cups almond flour
1 tbsp baking powder
¼ tsp salt
Directions:
Pour eggs and ghee into bread machine pan.
Add remaining ingredients.
Set bread machine to quick setting.
Allow bread machine to complete its cycle.
When the bread is done, remove bread machine pan from the bread machine.
Let cool slightly before transferring to a cooling rack.
The bread can be stored for up to 4 days on the counter and for up to 3 months in the freezer.
Nutrition:
Calories 167
Carbohydrates 2 g
Fats 16 g
Protein 5 g

42. Collagen Keto Bread

Preparation time: 5 minutes

Servings: 12

Ingredients:

½ cup collagen protein, unflavored grass-fed

6 tbsp almond flour

5 eggs

1 tbsp coconut oil, melted

1 tsp baking powder

1 tsp xanthan gum

¼ tsp Himalayan pink salt

Directions:

Pour all wet ingredients into bread machine bread pan.

Add dry ingredients to the bread machine pan.

Set bread machine to the gluten free setting

When the bread is done, remove bread machine pan from the bread machine.

Let cool slightly before transferring to a cooling rack.

The bread can be stored for up to 4 days on the counter and for up to 3 months in the freezer.

Nutrition:

Calories 77

Carbohydrates 6 g

Fats 14 g

Protein 5 g

43. Banana Cake Loaf

Preparation time: 4 minutes

Servings: 12

Ingredients:

1 ½ cups almond flour

1 tsp baking powder

½ cup butter

1 ½ cups erythritol

2 eggs

2 bananas, extra ripe, mashed

2 tsp whole milk

Directions:

Mix butter, eggs, and milk together in a mixing bowl.

Mash bananas with a fork and add in the mashed bananas.

Mix all dry ingredients together in a separate small bowl.

Slowly combine dry ingredients with wet ingredients.

Pour mixture into bread machine pan.

Set bread machine for bake.

When the cake is done remove from bread machine and transfer to a cooling rack.

Allow to cool completely before serving.

You can store your banana cake loaf bread for up to 5 days in the refrigerator.

Nutrition:

Calories 175

Carbohydrates 6 g

Fats 14 g

Protein 5 g

44. Almond Butter Brownies

Preparation time: 3 minutes
Servings: 14

Ingredients:
1 cup almond butter
2 tbsp cocoa powder, unsweetened
½ cup erythritol
1 egg
3 tbsp almond milk, unsweetened
Directions:
Beat egg and almond butter together in a mixing bowl.

Add in erythritol and cocoa powder.

If the mixture is too crumbly or dry, add in almond milk until you have a smooth consistency.

Pour mixture into bread machine pan.

Set bread machine to bake.

When done remove from bread machine and transfer to a cooling rack.

Cool completely before serving, You can store for up to 5 days in the refrigerator.

Nutrition:
Calories 141
Carbohydrates 3 g
Fats 12 g
Protein 5 g

45. Almond Butter Bread

Preparation time: 3 minutes
Servings: 8

Ingredients:
1 cup coconut almond butter, creamy
3 eggs
½ tsp baking soda
1 tbsp apple cider vinegar
Directions:
Combine all ingredients in a food processor.
When the mixture is smooth transfer to bread machine baking pan.
Set bread machine to bake.
When done baking, remove from the pan from your bread machine.
Allow to cool completely before slicing.
You can store for up to 5 days in the refrigerator.
Nutrition:
Calories 175
Carbohydrates 6 g
Fats 14 g
Protein 5 g

46. Cinnamon Cake

Preparation time: 7 minutes
Servings: 12

Ingredients:
½ cup erythritol
½ cup butter
½ tbsp vanilla extract
1 ¾ cups almond flour
1 ½ tsp baking powder
1 ½ tsp cinnamon
¼ tsp sea salt
1 ½ cup carrots, grated
1 cup pecans, chopped
Directions:
Grate carrots and place in a food processor.
Add in the rest of the ingredients, except the pecans, and process until well-incorporated.
Fold in pecans.
Pour mixture into bread machine pan.
Set bread machine to bake.
When baking is complete remove from bread machine and transfer to a cooling rack.
Allow to cool completely before slicing. (You can also top with a sugar-free cream cheese frosting, see recipe below).
You can store for up to 5 days in the refrigerator.
Nutrition:
Calories 350
Carbohydrates 8 g
Fats 34 g
Protein 7 g

47. Classic Gluten Free Bread

Preparation time: 5 minutes
Servings: 12

Ingredients:
½ cup butter, melted
3 tbsp coconut oil, melted
6 eggs
2/3 cup sesame seed flour
1/3 cup coconut flour
2 tsp baking powder
1 tsp psyllium husks
½ tsp xanthan gum
½ tsp salt
Directions:
Pour in eggs, melted butter, and melted coconut oil into your bread machine pan.
Add the remaining ingredients to the bread machine pan.
Set bread machine to gluten free.
When the bread is done, remove bread machine pan from the bread machine.
Let cool slightly before transferring to a cooling rack.
You can store your bread for up to 3 days.
Nutrition:
Calories 146
Carbohydrates 1.2 g
Fats 14 g
Protein 3.5 g

48. Gluten Free Chocolate Zucchini Bread

Preparation time: 5 minutes
Servings: 12

Ingredients:
1 ½ cups coconut flour
¼ cup unsweetened cocoa powder
½ cup erythritol
½ tsp cinnamon
1 tsp baking soda
1 tsp baking powder
¼ tsp salt
¼ cup coconut oil, melted
4 eggs
1 tsp vanilla
2 cups zucchini, shredded
Directions:
Shred the zucchini and use paper towels to drain excess water, set aside.
Lightly beat eggs with coconut oil then add to bread machine pan.
Add the remaining ingredients to the pan.
Set bread machine to gluten free.
When the bread is done, remove bread machine pan from the bread machine.
Let cool slightly before transferring to a cooling rack.
You can store your bread for up to 5 days.
Nutrition:
Calories 185
Carbohydrates 6 g
Fats 17 g
Protein 5 g

49. Not Your Everyday Bread

Preparation time: 7 minutes
Servings: 12

Ingredients:
2 tsp active dry yeast
2 tbsp inulin
½ cup warm water
¾ cup almond flour
¼ cup golden flaxseed, ground
2 tbsp whey protein isolate
2 tbsp psyllium husk finely ground
2 tsp xanthan gum
2 tsp baking powder
1 tsp salt
¼ tsp cream of tartar
¼ tsp ginger, ground
1 egg
3 egg whites
2 tbsp ghee
1 tbsp apple cider vinegar
¼ cup sour cream
Directions:
Pour wet ingredients into bread machine pan.
Add dry ingredients, with the yeast on top.
Set bread machine to basic bread setting.
When the bread is done, remove bread machine pan from the bread machine.
Let cool slightly before transferring to a cooling rack.
You can store your bread for up to 5 days.
Nutrition:
Calories 175
Carbohydrates 6 g
Fats 14 g
Protein 5 g

50. Pumpkin Bread

Preparation time: 5 minutes
Servings: 8

Ingredients:
6 eggs
8 tbsp butter, melted
2 cups almond flour
2 teaspoons baking powder
¼ teaspoon ground allspice
¼ teaspoon ground cloves
¼ teaspoon ground nutmeg
½ cup erythritol
½ cup pumpkin puree
1 tsp cinnamon
3 tbsps. sour cream
1 teaspoon vanilla
2 tbsp heavy cream
Directions:
In the bread machine pan add all the wet ingredients.
Then add the dry ingredients on top.
Set the bread machine to the gluten free bread setting.
When the bread is done, remove bread machine pan from the bread machine.
Let cool slightly before transferring to a cooling rack.
The bread can be stored for up to 5 days on the counter.
Nutrition:
Calories 220
Carbohydrates 14 g
Fats 21 g

51. Italian Blue Cheese Bread

Preparation time: 3 hours
Servings: 8

Ingredients:
1 teaspoon dry yeast
2 ½ cups almond flour
1 ½ teaspoon salt
1 tablespoon sugar
1 tablespoon olive oil
½ cup blue cheese
1 cup water
Directions:
Mix all the ingredients. Start baking.
Nutrition:
Carbohydrates 5 g
Fats 4.6 g
Protein 6 g
Calories 194

52. German Bread Linz

Preparation time: 3 ½ hours
Servings: 8

Ingredients
2 ¼ cups rye flour
2 ¼ cups almond flour
1 ¾ cups water + 2 eggs
2 teaspoons salt
2 tablespoons olive oil (odorless
2 teaspoons dry yeast
2 tablespoons honey
Directions:
Crack two eggs into a bowl, and add the rest of the ingredients.
Set the program for RYE BREAD or BASIC.
Bon Appetit!
Nutrition:
Carbohydrates 3.4 g
Fats 6 g
Protein 10.5 g
Calories 309

53. Apple Bread With Horseradish And Pistachios

Preparation time: 3 ½ hours

Servings: 8

Ingredients

3 cups almond flour

2 eggs

3 tablespoons grated horseradish

½ cup apple puree/applesauce

1 tablespoon sugar

4 tablespoons olive oil

½ cup chopped pistachios, peeled

1 teaspoon dried yeast

1 teaspoon salt

Directions:

Lightly beat eggs in a bowl. Pour in enough water to make 280 ml of liquid. Pour into a mold, and add olive oil.

Put in the flour, applesauce, horseradish, and half the pistachios. Add salt and sugar from different angles. Make a small groove in the flour and put in the yeast.

Bake on the BASIC program. After the final mixing of the dough, moisten the surface of the product with water and sprinkle with the remaining pistachios.

Let bread cool.

Nutrition:

Carbohydrates 2 g

Fats 10.9 g

Protein 7.7 g

Calories 291

54. Honey Bread With Cream And Coconut Milk

Preparation time: 3 ½ hours
Servings: 8

Ingredients
3 ¾ cups almond flour
1 ¾ cups bran meal
1 ¼ cups cream
1/3 cup coconut milk
2 tablespoons honey
2 tablespoons vegetable oil
2 teaspoons dry yeast
2 teaspoons salt
Directions:
Pour in the cream, coconut milk, ½ cup of water, honey, and vegetable oil.
Put in the flour and salt. Make a groove in the flour and put in the yeast.
Bake on the BASIC program.
Cool the bread and serve.
Nutrition:
Carbohydrates 4 g
Fats 8.6 g
Protein 8.1 g
Calories 348

55. Milk Almond Bread

Preparation time: 3 ½ hours
Servings: 8

Ingredients
1 ¼ cups milk
5 ¼ cups almond flour
2 tablespoons butter
2 teaspoons dry yeast
1 tablespoon sugar
2 teaspoons salt

Directions:

Pour the milk into the form and ½ cup of water. Add flour.

Put butter, sugar, and salt in different corners of the mold. Make a groove in the flour and put in the yeast.

Bake on the Basic program.

Cool the bread.

Nutrition:

Carbohydrates 5 g

Fats 4.5 g

Protein 10.1 g

Calories 352

56. Almond Bread With A Delicate Crust

Preparation time: 3 ½ hours
Servings: 8

Ingredients
1 ¼ cups milk
5 ¼ cups almond flour
2 tablespoons vegetable oil
2 tablespoons sour cream
2 teaspoons dried yeast
1 tablespoon sugar
2 teaspoons salt

Directions:
Pour the milk into the form and ½ cup of water, then add flour.

Put butter, sugar, and salt in different corners of the mold. Make a groove in the flour and add the yeast.

Bake on the Basic program.

After the final mixing of the dough, smear the surface of the product with sour cream.

Cool; serve; enjoy.

Nutrition:
Carbohydrates 4.5 g
Fats 4.9 g
Protein 8.9 g
Calories 344

57. Rice Bread

Preparation time: 3 ½ hours
Servings: 8

Ingredients
4 ½ cups almond flour
1 cup, rice, cooked
1 egg
2 tablespoons milk powder
2 teaspoons dried yeast
2 tablespoons butter
1 tablespoon sugar
2 teaspoons salt
Directions:
Pour 1 ¼ cups of water into the mold; add the egg.
Add flour, rice, and milk powder.
Put butter, sugar, and salt in different corners of the mold. Make a groove in the flour, and put in the yeast.
Bake on the Basic program.
When ready, cool the bread.
Nutrition:
Carbohydrates 5 g
Fats 4.2 g
Protein 9.6 g
Calories 328

58. Rice Bread With Soy Sauce

Preparation time: 3 ½ hours
Servings: 8

Ingredients
4 ½ cups almond flour
1 cup, rice, cooked
1 egg
2 tablespoons soy sauce
2 teaspoons dried yeast
2 tablespoons melted butter
1 tablespoon brown sugar
2 teaspoons salt
Directions:
Pour 1 ¼ cups of water, and soy sauce; add the egg.
Put in the flour and rice.
Put ghee, sugar, and salt in different corners of the mold. Make a groove in the flour, and put in the yeast.
Bake in "normal, medium crust" mode.
Bread is ready to eat when cooled.
Nutrition:
Carbohydrates 3.6 g
Fats 4.2 g
Protein 9.1 g
Calories 321

59. Bread With Chicken And Apricots

Preparation time: 2 hours
Servings: 6

Ingredients:
1 smoked chicken breast
2 cups of apricots
15 oz almond flour
15 oz rye flour
4 chopped cloves of garlic
2 onions
3 teaspoons dry yeast
1 cup of warm milk
2 tablespoons sugar
3 tablespoons olive oil
Sea salt
ground black pepper
Directions:
Soak the apricots in the warm water for 10 minutes and then cube them.
Chop the onions and fry until clear and golden brown and caramelized.
Cut the smoked chicken breast into small pieces and combine with the apricots.
Combine all the ingredients and mix well.
Pour some oil into a bread machine and place the dough into the bread maker. Cover the dough with the towel and leave for 1 hour.
Close the lid and turn the bread machine on the basic program.
Bake until the medium crust and after the bread is ready take it out and leave for few hours on a grate and only then slice.
Nutrition:
Carbohydrates 4.2 g
Fats 9 g
Protein 21 g
Calories 239

60. Bread With Turkey And Raisins

Preparation time: 3 hours
Servings: 8

Ingredients:
20 oz turkey
1 cup of raisins
2 big onions
2 cloves chopped garlic
1 cup of milk
25 oz almond flour
10 oz rye flour
3 teaspoons dry yeast
1 egg
3 tablespoons sunflower oil
1 teaspoon sugar
Himalayan salt
Directions:
Soak the raisins in the warm water for 10 minutes.
Boil the turkey meat with the salt on medium heat until soft. You can use
the turkey breast or fillet.
Blend the cooked and soft turkey meat using a food processor until it has a
smooth consistency.
Chop the onions and garlic and then fry them until clear and caramelized.
Combine the yeast with the warm water, mixing until smooth consistency.
Combine all the ingredients with the yeast, turkey, onions, raisins, garlic and
then mix and knead well.
Pour some oil into a bread machine and place the dough into the bread
maker. Cover the dough with the towel and leave for 1 hour.
Close the lid and turn the bread machine on the basic program.
Bake the bread until the medium crust and after the bread is ready take it
out and leave for 1 hour covered with the towel and only then you can slice
the bread.
Nutrition:
Carbohydrates 4.9 g
Fats 6.8 g
Protein 34 g
Calories 329

61. Bread With Beef And Peanuts

Preparation time: 3 hours
Servings: 8

Ingredients:
15 oz beef meat
5 oz Herbes de Provence
2 big onions
2 cloves chopped garlic
1 cup of milk
20 oz almond flour
10 oz rye flour
3 teaspoons dry yeast
1 egg
3 tablespoons sunflower oil
1 tablespoon sugar
Sea salt
ground black pepper
red pepper
Directions:
Sprinkle the beef meat with the Herbs de Provence, salt, black, and red pepper and marinate in bear for overnight.
Cube the beef and fry in a skillet or a wok on medium heat until soft (for around 20 minutes).
Chop the onions and garlic and then fry them until clear and caramelized.
Combine all the ingredients except for the beef and then mix well.
Combine the beef pieces and the dough and mix in the bread machine.
Close the lid and turn the bread machine on the basic program.
Bake the bread until the medium crust and after the bread is ready take it out and leave for 1 hour covered with the towel and only then you can slice the bread.
Nutrition:
Carbohydrates 4 g
Fats 42 g
Protein 27 g
Calories 369

62. Basic Sweet Yeast Bread

Preparation time: 3 hours
Servings: 8

Ingredients:
1 egg
¼ cup butter
1/3 cup sugar
1 cup milk
½ teaspoon salt
4 cups almond flour
1 tablespoon active dry yeast
After beeping:
fruits/ground nuts
Directions:
Add all of the ingredients to your bread machine, carefully following the instructions of the manufacturer (except fruits/ground nuts).
Set the program of your bread machine to BASIC/SWEET and set crust type to LIGHT or MEDIUM.
Press START.
Once the machine beeps, add fruits/ground nuts.
Wait until the cycle completes.
Once the loaf is ready, take the bucket out and let the loaf cool for 5 minutes.
Gently shake the bucket to remove loaf.
Transfer to a cooling rack, slice and serve.
Enjoy!
Nutrition:
Carbohydrates 2.7 g
Fats 7.6 g
Protein 8.8 g
Calories 338

63. Apricot Prune Bread

Preparation time: 3 hours
Servings: 8

Ingredients:
1 egg
4/5 cup whole milk
¼ cup apricot juice
¼ cup butter
1/5 cup sugar
4 cups almond flour
1 tablespoon instant yeast
¼ teaspoon salt
5/8 cup prunes, chopped
5/8 cup dried apricots, chopped
Directions:
Add all of the ingredients to your bread machine, carefully following the instructions of the manufacturer (except apricots and prunes).
Set the program of your bread machine to BASIC/SWEET and set crust type to LIGHT or MEDIUM.
Press START.
Once the machine beeps, add apricots and prunes.
Wait until the cycle completes.
Once the loaf is ready, take the bucket out and let the loaf cool for 5 minutes.
Gently shake the bucket to remove loaf.
Transfer to a cooling rack, slice and serve.
Enjoy!
Nutrition:
Carbohydrates 4 g
Fats 8.2 g
Protein 9 g
Calories 364

64. Citrus Bread

Preparation time: 3 hours
Servings: 8

Ingredients:
1 egg
3 tablespoons butter
1/3 cup sugar
1 tablespoon vanilla sugar
½ cup orange juice
2/3 cup milk
1 teaspoon salt
4 cup almond flour
1 tablespoon instant yeast
¼ cup candied oranges
¼ cup candied lemon
2 teaspoons lemon zest
¼ cup almond, chopped
Directions:
Add all of the ingredients to your bread machine, carefully following the
instructions of the manufacturer (except candied fruits, zest, and almond).
Set the program of your bread machine to BASIC/SWEET and set crust type
to LIGHT or MEDIUM.
Press START.
Once the machine beeps, add candied fruits, lemon zest, and chopped
almonds.
Wait until the cycle completes.
Once the loaf is ready, take the bucket out and let the loaf cool for 5
minutes.
Gently shake the bucket to remove loaf.
Transfer to a cooling rack, slice and serve.
Enjoy!
Nutrition:
Carbohydrates 4 g
Fats 9.1 g
Protein 9.8 g
Calories 404

65. Fruit Bread

Preparation time: 3 hours
Servings: 8

Ingredients:
1 egg
1 cup milk
2 tablespoons rum
¼ cup butter
¼ cup brown sugar
4 cups almond flour
1 tablespoon instant yeast
1 teaspoon salt
Fruits:
¼ cups dried apricots, coarsely chopped
¼ cups prunes, coarsely chopped
¼ cups candied cherry, pitted
½ cups seedless raisins
¼ cup almonds, chopped
Directions:
Add all of the ingredients to your bread machine, carefully following the instructions of the manufacturer (except fruits).
Set the program of your bread machine to BASIC/SWEET and set crust type to LIGHT or MEDIUM.
Press START.
Once the machine beeps, add fruits.
Wait until the cycle completes.
Once the loaf is ready, take the bucket out and let the loaf cool for 5 minutes.
Gently shake the bucket to remove loaf.
Transfer to a cooling rack, slice and serve.
Enjoy!
Nutrition:
Carbohydrates 5 g
Fats 10.9 g
Protein 10.8 g
Calories 441

66. Marzipan Cherry Bread

Preparation time: 3 hours
Servings: 8

Ingredients:
1 egg
¾ cup milk
1 tablespoon almond liqueur
4 tablespoons orange juice
½ cup ground almonds
¼ cup butter
1/3 cup sugar
4 cups almond flour
1 tablespoon instant yeast
1 teaspoon salt
½ cup marzipan
½ cup dried cherries, pitted
Directions:
Add all of the ingredients to your bread machine, carefully following the instructions of the manufacturer (except marzipan and cherry).
Set the program of your bread machine to BASIC/SWEET and set crust type to LIGHT or MEDIUM.
Press START.
Once the machine beeps, add marzipan and cherry.
Wait until the cycle completes.
Once the loaf is ready, take the bucket out and let the loaf cool for 5 minutes.
Gently shake the bucket to remove loaf.
Transfer to a cooling rack, slice and serve.
Enjoy!
Nutrition:
Carbohydrates 4.2 g
Fats 16.4 g
Protein 12.2 g
Calories 511

67. Ginger Prune Bread

Preparation time: 3 hours
Servings: 8

Ingredients:
2 eggs
1 cup milk
¼ cup butter
¼ cup sugar
4 cups almond flour
1 tablespoon instant yeast
1 teaspoon salt
1 cup prunes, coarsely chopped
1 tablespoon fresh ginger, grated
Directions:
Add all of the ingredients to your bread machine, carefully following the instructions of the manufacturer (except ginger and prunes).
Set the program of your bread machine to BASIC/SWEET and set crust type to LIGHT or MEDIUM.
Press START.
Once the machine beeps, add ginger and prunes.
Wait until the cycle completes.
Once the loaf is ready, take the bucket out and let the loaf cool for 5 minutes.
Gently shake the bucket to remove loaf.
Transfer to a cooling rack, slice and serve.
Enjoy!
Nutrition:
Carbohydrates 4 g
Fats 8.3 g
Protein 10.1 g
Calories 387

68. Marzipan Bread

Preparation time: 2 hours 10 minutes
Servings: 8

Ingredients:
4 eggs
½ cup butter
¾ cup sugar
1 tablespoon vanilla sugar
2 ½ cups almond flour
1 tablespoon baking powder
¼ cup almond, ground
½ cup marzipan, grated
Directions:
Add all of the ingredients to your bread machine, carefully following the instructions of the manufacturer (except marzipan).
Set the program of your bread machine to CAKE/SWEET and set crust type to LIGHT.
Press START.
Once the machine beeps, add marzipan.
Wait until the cycle completes.
Once the loaf is ready, take the bucket out and let the loaf cool for 5 minutes.
Gently shake the bucket to remove loaf.
Transfer to a cooling rack, slice and serve.
Enjoy!
Nutrition:
Carbohydrates 3 g
Fats 18.6 g
Protein 8.7 g
Calories 425

69. Lemon Fruit Bread

Preparation time: 3 hours
Servings: 8

Ingredients:
1 egg
1 cup milk
¼ cup butter
1/3 cup sugar
4 cups almond flour
1 tablespoon instant yeast
1 teaspoon salt
½ cup candied lemons
1½ teaspoon lemon zest, grated
½ cup raisins
½ cup cashew nuts
Directions:
Add all of the ingredients to your bread machine, carefully following the instructions of the manufacturer (except fruits, zest, and nuts).
Set the program of your bread machine to BASIC/SWEET and set crust type to LIGHT or MEDIUM.
Press START.
Once the machine beeps, add fruits, zest, and nuts.
Wait until the cycle completes.
Once the loaf is ready, take the bucket out and let the loaf cool for 5 minutes.
Gently shake the bucket to remove loaf.
Transfer to a cooling rack, slice and serve.
Enjoy!
Nutrition:
Carbohydrates 3.9 g
Fats 10.6 g
Protein 10 g
Calories 438
Total Fat 10.6 g, Saturated Fat 4.9 g, Cholesterol 38 mg, Sodium

70. Egg Liqueur Bread

Preparation time: 2 hours 10 minutes
Servings: 8

Ingredients:
3 eggs
½ cup egg liqueur
½ cup butter
½ cup sugar
1 tablespoon vanilla sugar
2 ½ cups almond flour
1 tablespoon baking powder
Directions:
Add all of the ingredients to your bread machine, carefully following the instructions of the manufacturer.
Set the program of your bread machine to CAKE/SWEET and set crust type to LIGHT.
Press START.
Wait until the cycle completes.
Once the loaf is ready, take the bucket out and let the loaf cool for 5 minutes.
Gently shake the bucket to remove loaf.
Transfer to a cooling rack, slice and serve.
Enjoy!
Nutrition:
Carbohydrates 5 g
Fats 14.3 g
Protein 6.7 g
Calories 349

71. Parmesan Bread

Preparation time: 3 hours
Servings: 10

Ingredients
2 ½ cups flour
1 ½ teaspoon fresh yeast
½ cup milk
1 tablespoon butter
2 tablespoons sugar
½ teaspoon salt
2 eggs at room temperature
2 teaspoons fresh rosemary, ground
3 tablespoons parmesan
2 cloves garlic
poppy seeds or sesame seeds for sprinkling
Directions:
It's simple. Combine all the ingredients for your bread maker in the bucket.
Dissolve yeast in warm milk in a saucepan and add in the last turn.
Run the program and do your own thing.
When the bread maker signals, add rosemary, parmesan, and garlic, passed through the garlic squeezer.
Make incisions and smear the top with milk; sprinkle with poppy seeds and/or parmesan.
Allow the bread to cool, turning it upside down or putting it on its side and covering with a towel.
Enjoy this delicious, homemade, and fragrant bread.
Nutrition:
Carbohydrates 3.2 g
Fats 4.6 g
Protein 7.6 g
Calories 212

72. Swiss Whole Meal Cheese Bread

Preparation time: 3 hours

Servings: 8

Ingredients

¾ cup warm water

1 tablespoon sugar

1 teaspoon salt

2 tablespoons green cheese

1 cup flour

9/10 cup flour whole-grain, finely ground

1 teaspoon yeast

1 teaspoon paprika

Directions:

Ingredients are listed in the order in which they are placed in the bread machine.

Add paprika at the signal.

The bread is gray, with a porous pulp. And, it does not become stale for a long time. It has a unique flavor, with very interesting cheese notes.

Nutrition:

Carbohydrates 5 g

Fats 1 g

Protein 4.1 g

Calories 118

73. Mustard Beer Bread

Preparation time: 3 hours
Servings: 8

Ingredients
1 ¼ cups dark beer
2 1/3 cups flour
¾ cup whole meal flour
1 tablespoon olive oil
3 teaspoons mustard seeds
1 ½ teaspoons dry yeast
1 teaspoon salt
2 teaspoons brown sugar
Directions:
Open a bottle of beer and let it stand for 30 minutes to get out the gas.
In a bread maker's bucket, add the beer, mustard seeds, butter, sifted flour, and whole meal flour.
From different angles in the bucket, put salt and sugar. In the center of the flour, make a groove and fill with the mustard seeds.
Start the baking program.
Nutrition:
Carbohydrates 4.2 g
Fats 1 g
Protein 4.1 g
Calories 118

Bread goes well with your salad and a great substitute if you want something light for lunch. You can eat breadsticks with your serve of keto pasta or grilled lemon chicken or how about grilled bacon and cheese sandwich with your favorite greens. Enjoy these mouthwatering bread recipes to satisfy your hunger.

74. Keto Flaxseed Honey Bread

Nutrition:
Calories: 96
Calories from fat: 36
Total Fat: 4 g
Total Carbohydrates: 5 g
Net Carbohydrates: 3 g
Protein: 8 g

Preparation Time: 10 minutes
Cooking Time: 20 minutes

Servings
18 slices
Ingredients
1 cup warm water
2 small eggs, lightly beaten
½ cup oat fiber
2/3 cup flaxseed meal
1.25 cup vital wheat gluten
1 tsp. salt
4 tbsp. swerve powdered sweetener
1 tsp. honey
½ tsp. xanthan gum
2 tbsps. Butter, unsalted
1 tbsp. dry active yeast
Directions
Pour the water on the bread bucket. e

Add the eggs, honey, erythritol, salt, oat fiber, flaxseed meal, wheat gluten, and xanthan in this order. Add softened butter and yeast.

Place back the bread bucket in your bread machine and close the lid. Select BASIC then select medium darkness on CRUST COLOR. Press START button and wait until the bread cooks.

Cool bread on a cooling rack before slicing.

Serve with grilled chicken or any of your favorite grilled meat. Note that nutrition info is only for the bread.

75. Keto Soft Pretzel Bread

Nutrition:

Calories: 217

Calories from fat: 162
Total Fat: 18 g
Total Carbohydrates: 3 g

Net Carbohydrates: 1 g
Protein: 11 g

Preparation Time: 1 hours 45 minutes
Cooking Time: 15 minutes

Servings

12 servings

Ingredients

3 cups mozzarella cheese

4 tbsps. Cream cheese

1 ½ cup almond flour

2 tsp. xanthan gum

2 small eggs

2 tsp. dried yeast

2 tbsps. Warm water

2 tbsps. Butter, melted and unsalted

1 tbsp. pretzel salt

Directions

Melt the mozzarella and cream cheese in the microwave for 3o seconds.

Dissolve the yeast in the warm water and 2 minutes to activate.

In a bowl, combine all the dry ingredients and mix well.

Using your bread bucket, pour the cheese mixture, the yeast mixture and the eggs.

Add the dry ingredient mixture and 1 tbsp. of butter.

Set the bread machine by selecting DOUGH, close the lid cover and press START button.

After kneading, take out the dough from the bread bucket and cut into 12 balls.

Preheat oven to 390 degrees F and prepare a lined cookie sheet.

Roll out each ball into long sticks and twist into a pretzel shape and place on the cookie sheet.

Brush the pretzel with the remaining 1 tbsp. butter and sprinkle with pretzel salt.

Bake for around 15 minutes or until it turns golden brown.

Serve with your favorite dip.

76. Keto Pepperoni Pizza

Nutrition:

Calories: 235

Calories from fat: 171
Total Fat: 19 g
Total Carbohydrates: 4 g

Net Carbohydrates: 2 g
Protein: 18 g

Preparation Time: 1 hour 30 minutes
Cooking Time: 20 minutes
Total Time: 1 hour 55 minutes

Servings

8 servings

Ingredients

Crust

2 cups mozzarella cheese, shredded

2 tbsps. Cream cheese

1 egg

¾ cup almond flour

Toppings

1 ½ cup mozzarella cheese, shredded

1 tsp. Italian seasoning

1/3 cup Rao's Marinara sauce

¼ cup pepperoni, sliced

Directions

To do the crust, melt the mozzarella and cream cheese in the microwave for 30 seconds. Transfer the cheese mixture in the bread bucket.

Add the egg then add the almond flour. Close the lid of the bread machine.

Turn the bread machine on by selecting DOUGH cycle and pressing the START button.

Wait for the bread machine ping before taking out the dough.

Preheat your oven to 425 degrees F. Spray your pizza pan with a non-stick spray and set aside.

Place your dough between two parchment paper and flatten it using a rolling pan into 12-inch round diameter.

Bake the dough for 10 minutes until lightly golden.

Remove crust from oven and spread the marinara sauce over the crust.

Sprinkle with mozzarella, and then arrange pepperoni on top.

Allow to bake for about 10 minutes more.

Cool down for about 5 minutes, then slice and serve.

77. Keto Chicken And Ranch Pizza

Nutrition:

Calories: 311

Calories from fat: 225
Total Fat: 25 g
Total Carbohydrates: 6 g

Net Carbohydrates: 4 g
Protein: 16 g

Preparation Time: 1 hour 40 minutes
Cooking Time: 15 minutes
Total Time: 1 hour 55 minutes

Servings

8 slices

Ingredients

Crust

2 cups mozzarella cheese, shredded

2 tbsps. Cream cheese

1 egg

¾ cup almond flour

1 tsp. salt

Ranch Sauce

½ cup mayonnaise

½ cup sour cream

¼ cup heavy cream

2 tbsps. White vinegar, distilled

2 cloves minced garlic

2 tbsps. Dill

1 tbsp. parsley

1 tsp. chives

1 tsp. onion powder

1 tsp. salt

Toppings

2 cups cheddar, shredded

1 cup grilled marinated chicken

6 strips bacon, fried and crumbled

2 tbsps. Chives, chopped

Directions

Prepare the crust, melt the mozzarella and cream cheese in the microwave for 30 seconds. Transfer the cheese mixture in the bread bucket.

Add the egg and salt, and then add the almond flour. Close the bread machine.

Turn the bread machine on by selecting DOUGH cycle then press the START button.

Wait for the bread machine to finish the dough cycle before taking out the dough.

Prepare the ranch sauce by combining all ingredients together and whisking well.

Preheat the oven at 425 degrees F and prepare a non-stick pizza pan. Set aside.

Shape your dough into a 12-inch diameter round size. Slide it in the oven and bake for 12 minutes or until light golden.

Spread 10 tablespoons of ranch over the crust and top with chicken, bacon and grated cheese. Pop back into the oven for 5 minutes or until cheese melts.

Sprinkle with chives before slicing and serving.

Notes: Ranch recipe yields about 20 tablespoons.

78. Keto Focaccia Squares

Nutrition:
Calories: 190
Calories from fat: 135
Total Fat: 15 g
Total Carbohydrates: 5 g
Net Carbohydrates: 3 g
Protein: 9 g

Preparation Time: 2 hours
Cooking Time: 15 minutes

Servings
9 squares
Ingredients
1 ½ cup mozzarella, shredded
1 oz. cream cheese, cubed
1 ½ cup almond flour, blanched
1 tbsp. baking powder
1 large egg, lightly beaten
Toppings
1 tbsp. rosemary leaves
½ tsp. coarse salt
Directions
Melt the mozzarella and cream cheese in the microwave for 30 seconds. Stir then microwave for another 40 seconds.
On you bread bucket, put the cheese, the egg, the almond flour, and the baking powder. Close the cover of the bread machine.
Start your bread machine and set it to DOUGH cycle. Press the START button to start the cycle.
Preheat your oven to 350 degrees Fahrenheit. Greased a 9-inch square pan.
Take the dough out and press on a square baking pan. Put dimples on your dough using your fingers.
Sprinkle your dough with rosemary leaves.
Place in the oven and bake for 15 to 17 minutes or until golden brown.
Cool the bread in a cooling rack for 15 minutes before cutting into nine squares.
Serve.

79. Keto Cajun Sandwich Loaf

Nutrition:

Calories: 35

Calories from fat: 9
Total Fat: 1 g
Total Carbohydrates: 5 g

Net Carbohydrates: 4 g
Protein: 1 g

Preparation Time: 10 minutes
Cooking Time: 2 hours

Servings

16 slices

Ingredients

½ cup water

¼ cup chopped onion

¼ cup chopped green bell peppers

2 tsp. fresh garlic, finely chopped

2 tsp. butter

2 cups almond flour

1 tbsp. sugar

1 tsp. Cajun seasoning

½ tsp. salt

1 tsp. active dry yeast

Directions

Put all the ingredients in the loaf bucket of your bread machine then close the cover.

Set your bread machine by selecting WHITE BREAD or BASIC cycle. Choose medium or dark color for CRUST COLOR setting. Press START.

Once your loaf bread is finish, place it in a cooling rack.

Slice and serve with ham and cheese to make a Cajun Ham and Cheese Sandwich.

80. Keto Flaxseed Sliced Bread

Nutrition:

Calories: 200

Calories from fat: 117
Total Fat: 13 g
Total Carbohydrates: 13 g

Net Carbohydrates: 3 g
Protein: 8 g

Preparation Time: 5 minutes
Cooking Time: 3 hours
5 minutes

Servings

15 slices

Ingredients

5 eggs

¼ cup coconut oil

2 tbsp. apple cider

½ tsp. salt

1 cup boiling water

1 tbsp. baking powder

2 tbsp. psyllium husk powder

2 cups flax seed flour

½ cup coconut flour

½ cup almond flour

2 tsp. dry active yeast

Directions

Put all the ingredients in your bread machine bucket as listed above. Pull down the lid of the bread machine.

Set your bread machine on BASIC cycle setting and select light on CRUST COLOR. Press the START button.

Once the cycle is complete, take out the loaf from the bread machine and cool on a cooling rack.

Slice and serve with cream cheese or any of your favorite spread.

81. Keto Hamburger Buns

Nutrition:

Calories: 57

Calories from fat: 45
Total Fat: 5 g
Total Carbohydrates: 2 g

Net Carbohydrates: 2 g
Protein: 1 g

Preparation Time: 2 hours 15 minutes
Cooking Time: 12 minutes

Servings

8 buns

Ingredients

1 large egg

½ cup almond milk, unsweetened

¼ cup water

2 tbsp. unsalted butter

1 tbsp. granulated sugar

¾ tsp. salt

2 ½ cups almond flour

1 1/8 tsp. active dry yeast

Directions

Put all ingredients in the order as listed above in your bread machine bucket.

Close the lid. Start your machine by selecting DOUGH cycle then press START.

Once the cycle is finished, transfer the dough on a floured surface. Cut the dough into 8-71 grams pieces. Form each piece into a ball and arranged on a greased lined baking sheet.

Flatten each ball into 1/2-inch thick then cover. Leave the dough to rise until the size doubles or after 30-35 minutes.

Preheat your oven at 400 degrees F. Pop the baking sheet into the oven and bake for 10-12 minutes or until golden brown.

Remove from oven and let it cool in a wire rack.

Serve with your Keto homemade burger or turkey slices.

82. Keto German Franks Bun

Nutrition:

Calories: 49

Calories from fat: 45
Total Fat: 5 g
Total Carbohydrates: 1 g

Net Carbohydrates: 1 g
Protein:2 g

Preparation Time: 2 hours
Cooking Time: 9 minutes
9 minutes

Servings

10 buns

Ingredients

1 ¼ cup almond milk, unsweetened, warmed

¼ cup sugar, granulated

1 small egg

2 tbsps. butter

¾ tsp. salt

3 ¾ cups almond flour

1 ¼ tsps. active dry yeast

Directions

Place all ingredients in your bread machine pan in the order listed above.

Close the lid of your bread machine, select DOUGH cycle and press START.

Once cycle is finish, transfer the dough into a floured surface. Cut the dough in 10 slices long.

Flatten the dough into 5 x 4 inches. Then tightly roll the dough to form a cylindrical shape size of 5 x 1 inch. Cover and let it rise for an hour or until the dough size doubles.

Preheat the oven at 350 degrees Fahrenheit. Arrange the dough in a greased baking sheet.

Place the baking sheet in the oven and bake for 9 minutes or until golden brown.

Cool then serve with your favorite franks.

83. Keto Beer Bread

Nutrition:

Calories: 118

Calories from fat: 90
Total Fat: 9
Total Carbohydrates: 3 g

Net Carbohydrates: 3 g
Protein: 6 g

Preparation Time: 10 minutes
Cooking Time: 2 hours

Servings

10 slices

Ingredients

10 oz. beer at room temperature

4 oz. American cheese, shredded

4 oz. Monterey Jack cheese, shredded

1 tbsp. sugar

1 ½ tsp. salt

1 tbsp. butter

3 cups almond flour

2.25 tsp. active dry yeast

Directions

In a microwave, combine beer and American cheese and warm for 20 seconds.

Transfer the beer mixture on the bread machine pan and add all the other ingredients as listed above.

Close the bread machine lid and select WHITE BREAD setting (or BASIC settingand press START button.

When the cycle ends, cool the bread on a cooling rack.

Slice and serve with a bowl of chili or beef stew.

84. Keto Monterey Jack Jalapeno Bread

Nutrition:

Calories: 47

Calories from fat: 27
Total Fat: 3 g
Total Carbohydrates: 3 g

Net Carbohydrates: 2 g
Protein: 2 g

Preparation Time: 15 minutes
Cooking Time: 2 hours

Servings

12 slices

Ingredients

1 cup water

3 tbsps. non-fat milk

1 ½ tbsps. sugar

1 ½ tsp. salt

1 ½ tbsps. butter, cubed

¼ cup Monterey Jack cheese, shredded

1 small jalapeno pepper

3 cups almond flour

2 tsp. active dry yeast

Directions

Remove the stem and seeds of the jalapeno and mince finely.

Add the ingredients in the bread machine pan as listed above.

Close the lid and select BASIC cycle and light or medium CRUST COLOR, then press START.

Once the cycle ends, transfer the loaf in a cooling rack before slicing.

Serve as a side dish for salad or your favorite main course.

85. Keto Pita Bread

Nutrition:

Calories: 37

Calories from fat: 27
Total Fat: 3 g
Total Carbohydrates: 2 g

Net Carbohydrates: 1 g
Protein: 1 g

Preparation Time: 3 hours 5 minutes
Cooking Time: 15 minutes

Servings

8 pieces

Ingredients

1 1/8 cups of warm water (1100 F

1 tsp. salt

1 tbsp. vegetable oil

1 ½ tsps. white sugar

3 cups almond flour

1 ½ tsp. active dry yeast

Directions

Place all ingredients in the bread machine bucket.

Pull down the cover and select DOUGH cycle setting before pressing START.

When machine beeps, transfer the dough to a floured surface.

Roll dough and stretch into a 12-inch long rope. Divide dough into 8 pieces then roll into a ball.

Flatten each ball into a 6-7-inch circle. Cover and let it raise for 30 minutes.

Preheat your oven at 500 degrees F. Place the pita bread on a wire rack and bake between 4-5 minutes or until it turns brown.

Remove from the oven and immediately cover with a damp kitchen towel until it turns soft.

Serve filled your favorite keto salad and meat.

86. Keto Rye Sandwich Bread

Nutrition:

Calories: 275

Calories from fat: 144
Total Fat: 16 g
Total Carbohydrates: 12

Net Carbohydrates: 8 g
Protein: 22 g

Preparation Time: 10 minutes
Cooking Time: 3 hours

Servings: 12 slices

Ingredients

2 ¼ cups warm water

6 tbsps. melted butter, unsalted

2 tsps. white sugar

1 ½ tsp. salt

1 tbsp. baking powder

¼ tsp. ground ginger

¼ cup granulated swerve

2 cups vital wheat gluten

2 cups super fine almond flour

¼ cup dark rye flour

4.5 tsps. active dry yeast

1 tbsp. caraway seeds

Directions

Place all ingredients in the bread machine bucket and close the lid.

Select the WHOLE WHEAT cycle in your bread machine setting and choose light color on CRUST COLOR. Press START.

When the cycle ends, remove the pan from the bread machine and transfer the loaf on a cooling rack.

Slice and make a pastrami or Rueben sandwich to serve.

87. Keto Cheese Loaf Bread

Nutrition:

Calories: 90

Calories from fat: 70
Total Fat: 7 g
Total Carbohydrates: 4 g

Net Carbohydrates: 4 g
Protein: 4 g

Preparation Time: 5 minutes
Cooking Time: 3 hours
5 minutes

Servings

Ingredients

1 1/3 cup warm water

4 tbsps. non-fat powder milk

4 tbsps. melted butter, unsalted

2 tbsps. brown sugar

1 tbsp. Italian seasoning

2 tsps. salt

4 cups almond flour

1 ½ tsp. active dry yeast

1 cup shredded cheese

Directions

Put all ingredients on the bread machine bucket in the order it is listed above. Do not include the shredded cheese.

Close the cover then select the BASIC cycle setting and light color on CRUST COLOR setting then press START.

Pause the bread machine after the final kneading and just before baking cycle. Open the lid and sprinkle the shredded cheese, then close the lid again and press START to continue.

Once the cycle is complete, remove the bucket from the machine and transfer the loaf onto a cooling rack.

Slice and serve plain or with spread.

88. Keto Orange Cranberry Bread

Nutrition:
Calories: 141
Calories from fat: 110
Total Fat: 12 g
Total Carbohydrates: 5 g
Net Carbohydrates: 4 g
Protein: 4 g

Preparation Time: 10 minutes
Cooking Time: 2 hours

Servings
10 slices
Ingredients
2 ¼ cup almond flour
1 tbsp. baking powder
¼ tsp. kosher salt
3 large eggs
1 ½ cup buttermilk
6 tbsp. canola oil
1 ½ cup brown sugar
½ tbsp. vanilla
½ tsp. nutmeg
¾ tsp. orange zest
2 tbsp. orange juice, fresh
1 cup fresh cranberries, chopped
Directions
Place all the ingredients in your bread machine bucket except for the cranberries.
Close the bread machine before selecting QUICK BREAD setting on your bread machine then press START.
Wait for the ping or the fruit and nut signal to open the lid and add the chopped cranberries. Close the lid again and press START to continue.
When the cycle finishes, transfer the loaf to a wire rack and let it cool.
Slice and serve with your favorite salad.

89. Low Carb Garlic Chia Bread Crackers

Servings: 4

Preparation time: 15 Minutes

Cooking Time: 30 Minutes

Ingredients

2 tablespoons chia seeds

1/2 cup chia or flax meal

1 tablespoon garlic powder

1 egg, whisked

1 teaspoon salt

Directions

Preheat your oven to 300 degrees.

In a bowl, mix together all ingredients until well blended; place the dough onto a flat surface and roll it out to 0.2-cm thickness and then cut into small squares.

Arrange the squares into a baking pan lined with parchment paper and bake for about 30 minutes. Remove from oven and let cool before serving with garlic dip. Enjoy!

Nutrition:

Calories: 123; Total Fat: 9 g; Carbs: 8 g; Dietary Fiber: 5 g; Sugars: 1 g; Protein: 6 g; Cholesterol: 104 mg; Sodium: 211 mg

90. Simple Low Carb Bread

Servings: 3 Servings

Preparation time: 5 Minutes

Cooking Time: 5 Minutes

Ingredients

1/4 cup golden flaxseed meal

1/4 cup almond flour

1/2 teaspoon kosher salt

1 teaspoon xanthan gum

1 teaspoon baking powder

1 scoop whey protein isolate

5 teaspoons erythritol

2 eggs

2 tablespoons butter melted & cooled

1 teaspoon apple cider vinegar

2 tablespoons sour cream

Directions

In a bowl, whisk together flaxseed meal, almond flour, xanthan gum, baking powder, whey protein and

In another bowl, whisk together sweetener and egg until the mixture is light and fluffy; whisk in butter and apple cider vinegar. Pour into the flour mix along with sour cream; whisk until well combined. Transfer the batter to a heatproof bowl. Place in the microwave and cook for about 5 minutes.

Serve the bread warm with butter.

Nutrition:

Calories: 237; Total Fat: 21 g; Carbs: 5 g; Dietary Fiber: 3 g; Sugars: 1 g; Protein: 6 g; Cholesterol: 79 mg; Sodium: 235 mg

91. Easy Low Carb Sandwich Bread

Servings: 12 Slices

Preparation time: 5 Minutes

Cooking Time: 25 Minutes

Ingredients

2 1/2 cups almond flour

3 teaspoons baking powder

1 tablespoons xanthan gum

2 cups whey protein

1 1/4 cups warm water

1/2 teaspoon salt

Directions

In a bowl, mix together dry ingredients until well combined; gradually whisk in warm water until dough comes together.

Line a loaf pan with paper and then press in dough. Bake for about 25 minutes at 375 degrees until the bread is golden brown and puffy. Remove from oven and let cool on the rack before slicing.

Enjoy!

Nutrition:

Calories: 197; Total Fat: 12 g; Carbs: 8 g; Dietary Fiber: 3 g; Sugars: 2 g; Protein: 18 g; Cholesterol: 3 mg; Sodium: 245 mg

92. Best Ever Keto Bread

Servings: 10 Slices

Total Time: 1 Hour 5 Minutes

Preparation time: 10 Minutes

Cooking Time: 55 Minutes

Ingredients

1½ cups blanched almond flour

3 egg whites

2½ tablespoons apple cider vinegar

5 tablespoons psyllium husk powder

1 teaspoon Celtic sea salt

2 teaspoons baking powder

7/8 cup boiling water

Directions

Preheat your oven to 350 degrees.

In a bowl, mix together almond flour, baking powder, salt and psyllium powder until well blended; whisk in vinegar and eggs until well combined. Whisk in warm water to form a soft dough.

Form about 5 mini loaves and arrange them on a greased sheet. Bake in the preheated oven for about 55 minutes. Remove the bread from oven and let cool on a rack before serving.

93. Easy Low Carb Bread

Servings: 1 Serving

Total Time: 5 Minutes

Preparation time: 2 Minutes

Cooking Time: 3 Minutes

Ingredients

3 tablespoons almond flour

1/2 teaspoon baking powder

A pinch of salt

1 large egg

1 tablespoon oil or melted butter

Directions

In a microwave safe bowl, mix all the ingredients until well combined; microwave for about 2 minutes. Remove and serve warm.

Nutrition:

Calories: 235; Total Fat: 20 g; Carbs: 5.7 g; Dietary Fiber: 3 g; Sugars: 1.5 g; Protein: 8 g; Cholesterol: 299 mg; Sodium: 321 mg

94. Garlicky & Rosemary Gluten-Free Bread

Servings: 10 Slices

Preparation time: 10 Minutes

Cooking Time: 45 Minutes

Ingredients

1/2 cup coconut flour

8 tablespoons butter

6 large eggs

1/2 teaspoon onion powder

1/2-1 teaspoon garlic powder

2 teaspoons dried rosemary

1 teaspoon baking powder

1/4 teaspoon salt

Directions

In a bowl, mix together all the dry ingredients until well combined.

In another bowl, whisk the eggs until light; whisk in melted butter until well combined and then slowly whisk into the dry ingredients until a soft dough forms.

Transfer the batter to a greased loaf pan and bake in a 350-degree oven for about 45 minutes. Remove from oven and let rest before serving.

Nutrition:

Calories: 147; Total Fat: 12.5 g; Carbs: 3.5 g; Dietary Fiber: 2 g; Sugars: 1 g; Protein: 4.6 g; Cholesterol: 318 mg; Sodium: 442 mg

95. Super Low Carb Flourless Bread

Servings: 12 Slices

Preparation time: 10 Minutes

Cooking Time: 21 Minutes

Ingredients

3 large eggs

1 cup cream cheese

1/4 cup parmesan cheese grated

2 cups mozzarella cheese grated

1 cup crushed pork rinds

herbs and spices

1 tablespoon baking powder

Directions

Preheat your oven to 375 degrees. Prepare a loaf pan by lining with parchment paper.

In a bowl, mix together dry ingredients until well combined.

In another bowl, whisk together wet ingredients until well blended; gradually whisk into the dry ingredients until a soft dough forms. Transfer the batter into a greased loaf pan and top with shredded cheese. Bake for about 20 minutes or until a tester inserted comes out clean.

Remove from oven and let cool before slicing to serve.

Nutrition:

Calories: 166; Total Fat: 13 g; Carbs: 1 g; Dietary Fiber: 0 g; Sugars: 0 g; Protein: 9 g; Cholesterol: 86 mg; Sodium: 294 mg

96. Simple Low Carb Bread

Servings: 16 Slices

Preparation time: 10 Minutes

Cooking Time: 40 Minutes

Ingredients

2/3 cup coconut flour

1 1/3 cup almond flour

1/2 teaspoon xanthan gum

1 teaspoon baking powder

1/2 teaspoon salt

3 tablespoons coconut oil, melted

1/2 cup butter, melted

6 large eggs

Directions

Preheat your oven to 355 degrees. Prepare a loaf pan by lining with parchment paper.

In a bowl, mix together dry ingredients until well combined.

In another bowl, whisk together wet ingredients until well blended; gradually whisk into the dry ingredients until a soft dough forms. Transfer the batter into a greased loaf pan and top with shredded cheese. Bake for about 40 minutes or until a tester inserted comes out clean.

Remove from oven and let cool before slicing to serve.

Nutrition:

Calories: 174; Total Fat: 15 g; Carbs: 5 g; Dietary Fiber2 9 g; Sugars: 0 g; Protein: 5 g; Cholesterol: 85 mg; Sodium: 163 mg

97. Low Carb Walnut Bread

Servings: 10 Slices

Preparation time: 10 Minutes

Cooking Time: 40 Minutes

Ingredients

1/2 cup coconut flour

2 tablespoons psyllium husk

1/2 teaspoon salt

1 tablespoon baking powder

2 tablespoons apple cider vinegar

4 tablespoons olive oil

4 eggs

1/2 cup boiling water

1 cup walnuts chopped

Directions

Preheat your oven to 350 degrees. Prepare a loaf pan by lining with parchment paper.

In a bowl, mix together dry ingredients until well combined.

In another bowl, whisk together wet ingredients until well blended; gradually whisk into the dry ingredients until a soft dough forms. Transfer the batter into a greased loaf pan and top with shredded cheese. Bake for about 40 minutes or until a tester inserted comes out clean.

Remove from oven and let cool before slicing to serve.

Nutrition:

Calories: 188; Total Fat: 16 g; Carbs: 7.3 g; Dietary Fiber: 4.3 g; Sugars: 2 g; Protein: 5 g; Cholesterol: 87 mg; Sodium: 200 mg

98. Rosemary Olive Bread

Servings: 10 Slices

Preparation time: 10 Minutes

Cooking Time: 35 Minutes

Ingredients

1/2 cup coconut flour

2 tablespoons psyllium husk

75grams chopped green olives

1 1/2 tablespoons dried rosemary

1 tablespoon baking powder

1/2 teaspoon salt

1 tablespoon apple cider vinegar

4 tablespoons olive oil

4 medium eggs

1/2 cups boiling water

Directions

Preheat your oven to 350 degrees. Prepare a loaf pan by lining with parchment paper.

In a bowl, mix together dry ingredients until well combined.

In another bowl, whisk together wet ingredients until well blended; gradually whisk into the dry ingredients until a soft dough forms. Transfer the batter into a greased loaf pan and top with shredded cheese. Bake for about 35 minutes or until a tester inserted comes out clean.

Remove from oven and let cool before slicing to serve.

Nutrition:

Calories: 123; Total Fat: 9 g; Carbs: 6 g; Dietary Fiber: 4.4 g; Sugars: 1 g; Protein: 3 g; Cholesterol: 96 mg; Sodium: 198 mg

99. Delicious Low Carb Challah Bread

Servings: 12 Slices

Preparation time: 10 Minutes

Cooking Time: 45 Minutes

Ingredients

3 tablespoons olive oil

1/4 cup heavy cream

1 ½ cup cream cheese

1 cup unflavored protein

2/3 cup vanilla protein

1/3 cup sweetener

1/4 cup butter

1/4 cup dried cranberries

4 eggs

1/2 teaspoon salt

1 teaspoon xanthan

1/2 of lemon zest

1/3 teaspoon baking soda

2 1/2 teaspoons baking powder

Directions

Preheat your oven to 320 degrees.

In a bowl, whisk eggs until light; stir in sweetener and then whisk in cream cheese along the remaining ingredients. Pour the mixture into a baking pan and bake for 45 minutes.

Nutrition:

Calories: 158; Total Fat: 13 g; Carbs: 2 g; Dietary Fiber: 0 g; Sugars: 1 g; Protein: 9 g; Cholesterol: 66 mg; Sodium: 241 mg

100. Healthy Keto Yogurt Buns

Servings: 4

Preparation time: 10 Minutes

Cooking Time: 35 Minutes

Ingredients

2 cup blanched almonds

2 teaspoons xanthan gum

2 teaspoons baking powder

4 tablespoons protein powder

1 teaspoon salt

4 tablespoons oil

4 eggs

2/3 cup yogurt

2 tablespoons water

Directions

Preheat your oven to 350 degrees. Prepare a baking sheet by lining with parchment paper and greasing with cooking spray.

In a bowl, mix together dry ingredients until well combined.

In another bowl, whisk together wet ingredients until well blended; gradually whisk into the dry ingredients until well blended. Cover and let rest for at least 1 hour. Roll the dough into balls and arrange them onto the prepared baking sheet. Bake for about 40 minutes or golden browned.

Nutrition:

Calories: 125; Total Fat: 10 g; Carbs: 2 g; Dietary Fiber: 1 g; Sugars: 0 g; Protein: 6 g; Cholesterol: 55 mg; Sodium: 112 mg

101. High Fiber Keto Bread Rolls

Servings: 4

Preparation time: 10 Minutes

Cooking Time: 40 Minutes

Ingredients

1 1/2 cups almond flour

3 tablespoons psyllium husk

3/4 cup potato or oat fiber

4 teaspoons baking powder

1/4 cup protein

1 cup Greek yogurt

2 tablespoons vinegar

2 tablespoons water

4 tablespoons oil

4 eggs

1 teaspoon salt

Directions

Preheat your oven to 350 degrees. Prepare a baking sheet by lining with parchment paper and greasing with cooking spray.

In a bowl, mix together dry ingredients until well combined.

In another bowl, whisk together wet ingredients until well blended; gradually whisk into the dry ingredients until well blended. Cover and let rest for at least 1 hour. Roll the dough into balls and arrange them onto the prepared baking sheet. Bake for about 40 minutes or golden browned.

Nutrition:

Calories: 177; Total Fat: 14 g; Carbs: 7 g; Dietary Fiber: 6 g; Sugars: 1 g; Protein: 11 g; Cholesterol: 115 mg; Sodium: 165 mg

102. Low Carb Tasty Bread

Servings: 12 Slices

Preparation time: 10 Minutes

Cooking Time: 50 Minutes

Ingredients

2 tablespoons coconut flour

1/4 teaspoon baking soda

1 teaspoon baking powder

1/2 teaspoon onion flakes

1/2 teaspoon garlic powder

1/2 teaspoon salt

3 eggs

1 tablespoon lemon juice

4 tablespoons unsweetened almond milk

3/4 cup almond butter

Directions

Preheat your oven to 300 degrees. Prepare a loaf pan by lining with parchment paper.

In a bowl, mix together dry ingredients until well combined.

In another bowl, whisk together wet ingredients until well blended; gradually whisk into the dry ingredients until a soft dough forms. Transfer the batter into a greased loaf pan and top with shredded cheese. Bake for about 50 minutes or until a tester inserted comes out clean.

Remove from oven and let cool before slicing to serve.

Nutrition:

Calories: 152; Total Fat: 12.9 g; Carbs: 5.4 g; Dietary Fiber: 2.7 g; Sugars: 1.8 g; Protein: 7.3 g; Cholesterol: 56 mg; Sodium: 142 mg

103. Best Keto Diet Bread

Servings: 12 Slices

Preparation time: 10 Minutes

Cooking Time: 15 Minutes

Ingredients

1 1/2 cup almond flour

2 tablespoons cream cheese

2 large egg beaten

2 1/2 cup shredded Mozzarella cheese

1 tablespoon erythritol

1 teaspoon active dry yeast

1 tablespoon baking powder

2 tablespoons sesame seeds

Directions

Preheat your oven to 400 degrees. Prepare a loaf pan by lining with parchment paper.

In a bowl, mix together dry ingredients until well combined.

In another bowl, whisk together wet ingredients until well blended; gradually whisk into the dry ingredients until a soft dough forms. Sprinkle with sesame seeds and then transfer the batter into a greased loaf pan and top with shredded cheese. Bake for about 15 minutes or until a tester inserted comes out clean.

Remove from oven and let cool before slicing to serve.

104. Farmers Low Carb Bread

Servings: 12 Slices

Preparation time: 30 Minutes

Cooking Time: 1 Hour 30 Minutes

Ingredients

1/3 cup ground psyllium husk

1 cup potato fiber

4 eggs

2 cups quark

2 tablespoons vinegar

1/2 cup boiling water

2 tablespoons baking powder

a pinch of salt

Directions

Preheat your oven to 300 degrees. Prepare a loaf pan by lining with parchment paper and greasing with cooking spray.

In a bowl, mix together dry ingredients until well combined.

In another bowl, whisk together wet ingredients until well blended; gradually whisk into the dry ingredients until well blended. Transfer the batter into a greased loaf pan. Bake for about 45 minutes or golden browned.

Remove from oven and let cool before slicing to serve.

Nutrition:

Calories: 133; Total Fat: 12 g; Carbs: 6 g; Dietary Fiber: 4 g; Sugars: 0 g; Protein: 2 g; Cholesterol: 199 mg; Sodium: 277 mg

105. Best Low Carb Buns

Servings: 5 Buns

Preparation time: 5 Minutes

Cooking Time: 15 Minutes

Ingredients

4 tablespoons almond flour

3 eggs

1/4 teaspoon xanthan gum

1 tablespoon parmesan cheese

1 cup cheddar cheese

Directions

In a large bowl, whisk the eggs; whisk in the remaining ingredients and then add about five spoonfuls onto a baking sheet that is lined with parchment paper. Bake for about 12 minutes at 350 degrees. Broil for about 3 minutes or until lightly browned.

Nutrition:

Calories: 119; Total Fat: 10.2 g; Carbs: 0.7 g; Dietary Fiber: 0.6 g; Sugars: 0 g; Protein: 7.2 g; Cholesterol: 187 mg; Sodium: 166 mg

106. Low Carb Blueberry Bread

Servings: 12 Slices

Preparation time: 10 Minutes

Cooking Time: 1 Hour 15 Minutes

Ingredients

For the Bread:

2 tablespoons sour cream

9 tablespoons melted butter

6 eggs

2 tablespoons heavy whipping cream

2/3 cup Monk fruit

3/4 cup fresh blueberries

10 tablespoons coconut flour

1/2 teaspoon cinnamon

1½ teaspoon baking powder

½ teaspoon salt

1½ teaspoon vanilla

For the Icing:

2 tablespoons Monk fruit Powdered

1/4 teaspoon lemon zest

dash of vanilla

1 tablespoon heavy whipping cream

1 teaspoon butter melted

Directions

Preheat your oven to 350 degrees. Prepare a loaf pan by lining with parchment paper and greasing with cooking spray.

In a bowl, mix together dry ingredients until well combined.

In another bowl, whisk together wet ingredients until well blended; gradually whisk into the dry ingredients until well blended. Transfer the batter into a greased loaf pan. Bake for about 65 minutes or golden browned.

Make the icing by mixing all ingredients until smooth; drizzle over the bread to serve.

Nutrition:

Calories: 155; Total Fat: 13 g; Carbs: 4 g; Dietary Fiber: 2 g; Sugars: 1 g; Protein: 3 g; Cholesterol: 111 mg; Sodium: 220 mg

107. Low Carb Orange & Cranberry Bread

Servings: 12 Slices

Preparation time: 15 Minutes

Cooking Time: 55 Minutes

Ingredients

9 tablespoons coconut flour

2/3 cup powdered sweetener

2 tablespoons sour cream

1 teaspoon vanilla

1 1/2 teaspoons orange extract

9 tablespoons melted butter

1 egg yolk

5 eggs

1 1/2 teaspoons baking powder

1/4 teaspoon salt

3 tablespoons powdered sweetener

1 cup chopped fresh cranberries

For the Glaze:

1 tablespoon heavy whipping cream

2 tablespoons powdered sweetener

1/2 tablespoon butter, melted

Directions

Preheat your oven to 350 degrees. Prepare a loaf pan by lining with parchment paper and greasing with cooking spray.

In a bowl, whisk together butter, eggs, egg yolks, vanilla extract, orange extract, sour cream, sweetener until well combined; whisk in coconut flour, salt and baking powder until well combined. Fold the cranberries into the batter and spoon the batter into the pan. Bake for about 55 minutes.

Meanwhile, in a bowl, whisk together melted butter, sweetener and heavy cream until well blended; pour over the hot bread and serve.

Nutrition:

Calories: 139; Total Fat: 12 g; Carbs: 3 g; Dietary Fiber: 1 g; Sugars: 1 g; Protein: 3 g; Cholesterol: 109 mg; Sodium: 168 mg

108. Delicious Low Carb Rolls

Servings: 4

Preparation time: 10 Minutes

Cooking Time: 20 Minutes

Ingredients

2 eggs

1/4 cup cream cheese

1/4 cup grated Parmesan cheese

1 ½ cup shredded Mozzarella cheese

1 ⅓ cup blanched almond flour

1 ½ teaspoons baking powder

Directions

Preheat your oven to 350 degrees. Prepare a muffin pan by lining with parchment paper and greasing with cooking spray.

In a bowl, mix together dry ingredients until well combined.

In another bowl, whisk together wet ingredients until well blended; gradually whisk into the dry ingredients until well blended. Form the balls from the dough and then roll each into grated parmesan cheese until well coated. Press three balls into each muffin cup and bake for about 20 minutes.

Nutrition:

Calories: 283; Total Fat: 12 g; Carbs: 4 g; Dietary Fiber: 2 g; Sugars: 1 g; Protein: 16 g; Cholesterol: 202 mg; Sodium: 110 mg

109. Simple And Quick Keto Muffins

Servings: 4

Preparation time: 5 Minutes

Cooking Time: 5 Minutes

Ingredients

1 tablespoon coconut flour

1/2 tablespoon melted coconut oil

1 egg beaten

1 tablespoon milk

1/8 teaspoon vanilla extract

1/2 teaspoon baking powder

1/4 teaspoon honey

1 pinch sea salt

Directions

Preheat your oven to 350 degrees.

In a bowl, mix together dry ingredients until well combined.

In another bowl, whisk together wet ingredients until well blended; gradually whisk into the dry ingredients until well blended. Transfer the batter to a ramekin and bake for about 15 minutes or golden browned.

Remove from oven and let cool before slicing to serve.

Nutrition:

Calories: 200; Total Fat: 12 g; Carbs: 5 g; Dietary Fiber: 2.5 g; Sugars: 1 g; Protein: 8 g; Cholesterol: 198 mg; Sodium: 413 mg

110. Cheddar Veggie Low Carb Bread

Servings: 10 Slices

Preparation time: 5 Minutes

Cooking Time: 30 Minutes

Ingredients

3 1/2 tablespoon coconut flour

3/4 cup chopped broccoli florets

1 cup shredded cheddar cheese

2 teaspoon baking powder

5 eggs beaten

1 teaspoon salt

Directions

Preheat your oven to 350 degrees. Prepare a loaf pan by lining with parchment paper and greasing with cooking spray.

In a bowl, mix together all ingredients until well combined. Transfer the batter into a greased loaf pan. Bake for about 45 minutes or golden browned.

Remove from oven and let cool before slicing to serve.

Nutrition:

Calories: 90; Total Fat: 6 g; Carbs: 11 g; Dietary Fiber: 1 g; Sugars: 0 g; Protein: 6 g; Cholesterol: 93 mg; Sodium: 342 mg

111. Crunchy Super Seed Bread

Servings: 16 slices

Preparation Time: 10 minutes

Cooking Time: 1 hour

Ingredients

1 1/2 cups pumpkin seeds raw (divided), 1 cup processed to form a coarse flour

1/2 cup flax seeds

1 cup sunflower seeds

1/2 cup chia seeds

1/2 cup flax seeds

1/2 cup whole psyllium husks

1 teaspoon pink sea salt

1 pinch r stevia

3 tablespoons extra virgin olive oil

1 1/2 cups Luke warm water

Directions

Start by setting your oven to 350 degrees F. Line a large loaf pan with parchment paper then set it aside.

Combine the pumpkin seed flour with all the other seeds including the remaining pumpkin seeds, psyllium husks, stevia and salt.

 Pour in the water, little by little, followed by the olive oil and mix until the dough thickens and is well combined. Scoop the dough into the prepared loaf pan, shaping it well using the back of a serving spoon and bake for 45 minutes. Check for readiness by inserting a toothpick at the center.

Remove from oven and gently flip it onto a baking sheet. Gently pull out the loaf pan and return the bread to the oven to bake for 15 more minutes. This will give the bread a beautiful crust.

   You will know that your loaf is perfectly done when you lightly tap on it and it sounds hollow. Transfer to a cooling rack and slice when completely cool.

Nutrition:

Calories: 153; Total Fat: 6g; Carbs: 2g; Dietary Fiber8 g; Protein: 7 g; Cholesterol: 0.73 mg; Sodium: 188mg

112. Ground Beef Pinwheels With Mushroom Sauce

Serving: 5
Preparation Time: 20 minutes
Cooking Time: 25 minutes

Ingredients
Meat:
1 pound ground beef
1/2 onion, chopped
1 clove garlic, minced
1/4 teaspoon ground black pepper
Pastry:
2 cups all-purpose flour
4 teaspoons baking powder
1 teaspoon salt
1/2 cup shortening
3/4 cup milk
Mushroom Sauce:
2 (10.75 ouncecans cream of mushroom soup
1 (10.75 ouncecan milk
Direction
Preheat oven to 400 degrees F (200 degrees C).

Heat a large skillet over medium-high heat. Cook and stir beef in the hot skillet until a bit of the fat renders, 2 to 3 minutes; add onion, garlic, and black pepper. Continue to cook and stir the beef mixture until the beef is browned completely, 3 to 5 minutes more.

Combine flour, baking powder, and salt in a large bowl. Cut shortening into the flour mixture with a pastry cutter or fork. Slowly pour 3/4 cup milk into the mixture while stirring with a fork to form a soft dough; knead 8 to 10 times and roll out into a 12x8-inch rectangle.

Spread the beef mixture in an even layer onto the pastry rectangle to cover, leaving one of the longer edges clear. Begin with longer end not left clear and roll pastry and filling tightly into a cylinder, pinching the edge left clear to seal.

Use a thread to cut cylinder into ten 1 1/2-inch slices; arrange pinwheels onto a baking sheet.

Bake in preheated oven until pastry is no longer doughy, 15 to 20 minutes.

Stir cream of mushroom soup and 1 can of milk together in a saucepan; bring to a simmer and cook until hot, 2 to 3 minutes. Spoon over the baked pinwheels.

Nutrition:

Calories: 692 calories

Total Fat: 41 g

Cholesterol: 65 mg

Sodium: 1736 mg

Total Carbohydrate: 54.3 g

Protein: 25.9 g

113. Herb Biscuits

Serving: 8
Preparation Time: 10 minutes
Cooking Time: 12 minutes

Ingredients

1 (12 ouncepackage refrigerated buttermilk biscuit dough

1/2 cup melted butter

1 1/2 teaspoons dried parsley

1 1/2 teaspoons dried dill weed

1/4 teaspoon dried minced onion

Direction

In a medium bowl, blend melted butter with the dried parsley, dill weed, and onion flakes.

Cut buttermilk biscuits into quarters. Roll each biscuit quarter in herb butter. Place in 8 inch cake pan, with pieces touching. Pour remaining butter over biscuits.

Bake in a 425 degree F (220 degrees Coven for 12 minutes. Serve warm.

Nutrition:

Calories: 238 calories

Total Fat: 17.2 g

Cholesterol: 31 mg

Sodium: 502 mg

Total Carbohydrate: 18.4 g

Protein: 3 g

114. Herb Buttermilk Biscuits

Serving: 12
Preparation Time: 20 minutes
Cooking Time: 8 minutes

Ingredients

2 cups sifted all-purpose flour

1 tablespoon baking powder

1 pinch salt

1 1/2 teaspoons white sugar

1 1/2 teaspoons dried thyme

1 1/2 teaspoons dried savory

1 teaspoon kelp powder

1 tablespoon dried parsley

1 tablespoon dried basil

1/3 cup unsalted butter, softened

3/4 cup buttermilk

Direction

Preheat oven to 450 degrees F (230 degrees C). Whisk together the flour, baking powder, salt, sugar, thyme, savory, kelp, parsley, and basil in a large bowl.

Cut in the butter with a knife or pastry blender until the mixture resembles coarse crumbs. Drizzle the buttermilk slowly over the flour mixture while tossing lightly with a fork, just until the flour mixture is moistened. Turn the dough out onto a floured board, and knead 4 to 5 times. Pat the dough into a circle, 3/4 inch thick, and cut biscuits with a 2 inch cookie cutter. Place biscuits 2 inches apart on a baking sheet.

Bake in the preheated oven until golden brown, about 8 minutes. Serve warm.

Nutrition:

Calories: 133 calories

Total Fat: 5.5 g

Cholesterol: 14 mg

Sodium: 147 mg

Total Carbohydrate: 18 g

Protein: 2.9 g

115. Herman Biscuits

Serving: 12
Preparation Time: 15 minutes
Cooking Time: 30 minutes

Ingredients

1 cup Herman Sourdough Starter

1 cup all-purpose flour

1/4 teaspoon baking soda

2 teaspoons baking powder

1/4 teaspoon salt

1/4 cup vegetable oil

Direction

Bring Herman Starter to room temperature.

Stir together flour, baking soda, baking powder and salt.

Stir flour mixture and oil into Herman Starter. It will form a soft dough.

On a lightly floured surface knead dough until smooth. Pinch off small pieces of dough and shape into balls OR roll dough out and cut with a biscuit cutter. Place biscuits onto a greased baking sheet, cover and let rise in a warm place for 1 hour.

Preheat oven to 350 degrees F (175 degrees C).

Bake in biscuits in the preheat oven for about 30 minutes or until golden. Serve warm.

Nutrition:

Calories: 79 calories

Total Fat: 4.7 g

Cholesterol: 0 mg

Sodium: 156 mg

Total Carbohydrate: 8.2 g

Protein: 1.1 g

116. Highrise Buttermilk Biscuits

Serving: 9
Preparation Time: 30 minutes
Cooking Time: 14 minutes

Ingredients
4 cups cake flour
2 1/2 tablespoons aluminum-free baking powder
2 teaspoons salt
1/2 cup cold unsalted butter, cut into small chunks
1 1/3 cups buttermilk, or more as needed
1 tablespoon salted butter, melted
Direction
Preheat oven to 500 degrees F (260 degrees C).
Mix flour, baking powder, and salt together in the bowl of a stand mixer with
a paddle attachment. Add unsalted butter and mix at medium speed until
well incorporated and the mixture resembles wet sand, about 4 minutes.
Remove the bowl from the mixer and fold in buttermilk until dough sticks
together.
Dump dough onto a flour work surface; pat into a rectangle. Pat remaining
dry crumbs into the mixture by hand.
Cut dough in half with a floured bench knife; stack cut halves on top of each
other. Press layers together to about 1 1/2-inch thickness, shaping a long
rectangle as you go. Repeat 3 to 5 times.
Cut dough into 8 even squares with the bench knife. Cut off uneven edges
and put these scraps to the side; clean cuts on all sides will encourage rise.
Pat scraps together to make 1 odd-shaped ninth biscuit.
Place biscuits close together in a 9-inch square pan and brush with melted
salted butter. Place pan on top of the warm stove for 10 to 15 minutes to
rise.
Bake biscuits in the preheated oven, checking halfway through bake time,
until tops are golden brown and a toothpick inserted into the center comes
out clean, 14 to 18 minutes.
Nutrition:
Calories: 349 calories
Total Fat: 12.4 g
Cholesterol: 32 mg
Sodium: 973 mg
Total Carbohydrate: 52.5 g
Protein: 6.5 g

Chapter 2. Vegetable Loaves

117. Cheesy Broccoli Bread 2

Preparation time: 10 minutes

Cooking time: 30 minutes

Servings: 4

Ingredients:

5 eggs, whisked

2 teaspoons baking powder

1 cup cheddar, shredded

1 cup broccoli florets, separated

4 tablespoons coconut flour

Cooking spray

Directions:

In a bowl, mix all the ingredients except the cooking spray and stir really well.

Pour the batter in a loaf pan greased with cooking spray and bake at 350 degrees F for 30 minutes.

Cool the bread down, slice and serve.

Nutrition: calories 123, fat 6, fiber 1, carbs 3, protein 6

118. Keto Spinach Bread

Preparation time: 10 minutes

Cooking time: 30 minutes

Servings: 10

Ingredients:

½ cup spinach, chopped

1 tablespoon olive oil

1 cup water

3 cups almond flour

A pinch of salt and black pepper

1 tablespoon stevia

1 teaspoon baking powder

1 teaspoon baking soda

½ cup cheddar, shredded

Directions:

In a bowl, mix the flour, with salt, pepper, stevia, baking powder, baking soda and the cheddar and stir well.

Add the remaining ingredients, stir the batter really well and pour it into a lined loaf pan.

Cook at 350 degrees F for 30 minutes, cool the bread down, slice and serve.

Nutrition: calories 142, fat 7, fiber 3, carbs 5, protein 6

119. Cinnamon Asparagus Bread

Preparation time: 10 minutes

Cooking time: 45 minutes

Servings: 8

Ingredients:

1 cup stevia

¾ cup coconut oil, melted

1 and ½ cups almond flour

2 eggs, whisked

A pinch of salt

1 teaspoon baking soda

1 teaspoon cinnamon powder

2 cups asparagus, chopped

Cooking spray

Directions:

In a bowl, mix all the ingredients except the cooking spray and stir the batter really well.

Pour this batter into a loaf pan greased with cooking spray and bake at 350 degrees F for 45 minutes, cool the bread down, slice and serve.

Nutrition: calories 165, fat 6, fiber 3, carbs 5, protein 6

120. Kale And Cheese Bread

Preparation time: 10 minutes

Cooking time: 1 hour

Servings: 8

Ingredients:

2 cups kale, chopped

1 cup warm water

1 teaspoon baking powder

1 teaspoon baking soda

2 tablespoons olive oil

2 teaspoons stevia

1 cup parmesan, grated

3 cups almond flour

A pinch of salt

1 egg

2 tablespoons basil, chopped

Directions:

In a bowl, mix the flour, salt, parmesan, stevia, baking soda and baking powder and stir.

Add the rest of the ingredients gradually and stir the dough well.

Transfer it to a lined loaf pan, cook at 350 degrees F for 1 hour, cool down, slice and serve.

Nutrition: calories 231, fat 7, fiber 2, carbs 5, protein 7

121. Beet Bread

Preparation time: 1 hour and 10 minutes

Cooking time: 35 minutes

Servings: 6

Ingredients:

1 cup warm water

3 and ½ cups almond flour

1 and ½ cups beet puree

2 tablespoons olive oil

A pinch of salt

1 teaspoon stevia

1 teaspoon baking powder

1 teaspoon baking soda

Directions:

In a bowl, mix the flour with the water and beet puree and stir well.

Add the rest of the ingredients, stir the dough well and pour it into a lined loaf pan.

Leave the mix to rise in a warm place for 1 hour, and then bake the bread at 375 degrees F for 35 minutes.

Cool the bread down, slice and serve.

Nutrition: calories 200, fat 8, fiber 3, carbs 5, protein 6

122. Keto Celery Bread

Preparation time: 2 hours and 10 minutes

Cooking time: 35 minutes

Servings: 6

Ingredients:

½ cup celery, chopped

3 cups almond flour

1 teaspoon baking powder

1 teaspoon baking soda

A pinch of salt

2 tablespoons coconut oil, melted

½ cup celery puree

Directions:

In a bowl, mix the flour with salt, baking powder and baking soda and stir.

Add the rest of the ingredients, stir the dough well, cover the bowl and keep in a warm place for 2 hours.

Transfer the dough to a lined loaf pan and cook at 400 degrees F for 35 minutes.

Cool the bread down, slice and serve.

Nutrition: calories 162, fat 6, fiber 2, carbs 6, protein 4

123. Easy Cucumber Bread

Preparation time: 10 minutes

Cooking time: 50 minutes

Servings: 6

Ingredients:

1 cup erythritol

1 cup coconut oil, melted

1 cup almonds, chopped

1 teaspoon vanilla extract

A pinch of salt

A pinch of nutmeg, ground

½ teaspoon baking powder

A pinch of cloves

3 eggs

1 teaspoon baking soda

1 tablespoon cinnamon powder

2 cups cucumber, peeled, deseeded and shredded

3 cups coconut flour

Cooking spray

Directions:

In a bowl, mix the flour with cucumber, cinnamon, baking soda, cloves, baking powder, nutmeg, salt, vanilla extract and the almonds and stir well.

Add the rest of the ingredients except the coconut flour, stir well and transfer the dough to a loaf pan greased with cooking spray.

Bake at 325 degrees F for 50 minutes, cool the bread down, slice and serve.

Nutrition: calories 243, fat 12, fiber 3, carbs 6, protein 7

124. Red Bell Pepper Bread

Preparation time: 10 minutes

Cooking time: 30 minutes

Servings: 12

Ingredients:

1 and ½ cups red bell peppers, chopped

1 teaspoon baking powder

1 teaspoon baking soda

2 tablespoons warm water

1 and ¼ cups parmesan, grated

A pinch of salt

4 cups almond flour

2 tablespoons ghee, melted

1/3 cup almond milk

1 egg

Directions:

In a bowl, mix the flour with salt, parmesan, baking powder, baking soda and the bell peppers and stir well.

Add the rest of the ingredients and stir the bread batter well.

Transfer it to a lined loaf pan and bake at 350 degrees F for 30 minutes.

Cool the bread down, slice and serve.

Nutrition: calories 100, fat 5, fiber 1, carbs 4, protein 4

125. Tomato Bread

Preparation time: 1 hour and 10 minutes

Cooking time: 35 minutes

Servings: 12

Ingredients:

6 cups almond flour

½ teaspoon basil, dried

¼ teaspoon rosemary, dried

1 teaspoon oregano, dried

½ teaspoon garlic powder

2 tablespoons olive oil

2 cups tomato juice

½ cup tomato sauce

1 teaspoon baking powder

1 teaspoon baking soda

3 tablespoons swerve

Directions:

In a bowl, mix the flour with basil, rosemary, oregano and garlic and stir.

Add the rest of the ingredients and stir the batter well.

Pour into a lined loaf pan, cover and keep in a warm place for 1 hour.

Bake the bread at 375 degrees F for 35 minutes, cool down, slice and serve.

Nutrition: calories 102, fat 5, fiber 3, carbs 7, protein 4

126. Herbed Keto Bread

Preparation time: 1 hour and 30 minutes

Cooking time: 40 minutes

Servings: 8

Ingredients:

3 cups coconut flour

1 teaspoon baking powder

1 teaspoon baking soda

2 teaspoons stevia

1 and ½ cups warm water

½ teaspoon basil, dried

1 teaspoon oregano, dried

½ teaspoon thyme, dried

½ teaspoon marjoram, dried

2 tablespoons olive oil

Directions:

In a bowl, mix the flour with baking powder, baking soda, stevia, basil, oregano, thyme, and the marjoram and stir.

Add the remaining ingredients, mix the dough, cover and keep in a warm place for 1 hour and 30 minutes.

Transfer the dough to a floured working surface and knead it again for 2-3 minutes.

Transfer to a lined loaf pan and bake at 400 degrees F for 40 minutes.

Cool the bread down before serving.

Nutrition: calories 200, fat 7, fiber 3, carbs 5, protein 6

127. Olive Bread

Preparation time: 10 minutes

Cooking time: 45 minutes

Servings: 12

Ingredients:

1 teaspoon baking powder

1 and ½ cups warm water

A pinch of salt

3 cups almond flour

1 cup black olives, pitted and sliced

Directions:

In a large bowl, mix all the ingredients and knead until you obtain a dough.

Cover the bowl, keep the dough in a warm place for 40 minutes and then transfer it to a lined round loaf pan.

Bake the bread at 400 degrees F for 40 minutes, cool it down, slice and serve.

Nutrition: calories 222, fat 7, fiber 3, carbs 5, protein 6

128. Green Olive Bread

Preparation time: 10 minutes

Cooking time: 45 minutes

Servings: 10

Ingredients:

3 cups almond flour

A pinch of salt

½ teaspoon baking powder

1 and ½ cups warm water

3 tablespoons rosemary, chopped

½ cup green olives, pitted and chopped

A pinch of salt and black pepper

Directions:

In a bowl, mix the flour with salt, rosemary and baking powder and stir.

Add the rest of the ingredients, mix the dough well and transfer it to a lined loaf pan.

Bake at 400 degrees F for 45 minutes, cool down, slice and serve.

Nutrition: calories 204, fat 12, fiber 4, carbs 5, protein 7

129. Delicious Eggplant Bread

Preparation time: 10 minutes

Cooking time: 1 hour

Servings: 12

Ingredients:

4 eggs, whisked

1 cup erythritol

½ cup ghee, melted

½ cup coconut oil, melted

2 cups eggplant, peeled and grated

1 tablespoon vanilla extract

2 cups almond flour

1 and ½ teaspoon cinnamon powder

¼ teaspoon nutmeg, ground

½ teaspoon baking powder

1 teaspoon baking soda

A pinch of salt

½ cup pine nuts

Cooking spray

Directions:

In a bowl, mix the flour with cinnamon, nutmeg, baking powder, baking soda, salt, pine nuts and the vanilla and stir.

Add the rest of the ingredients except the cooking spray, mix the batter well and pour into a loaf pan greased with the cooking spray.

Cook at 350 degrees F for 1 hour, cool down, slice and serve.

Nutrition: calories 200, fat 7, fiber 3, carbs 5, protein 6

130. Great Blackberries Bread

Preparation time: 10 minutes

Cooking time: 1 hour

Servings: 10

Ingredients:

2 cups almond flour

½ cup stevia

1 and ½ teaspoons baking powder

1 teaspoon baking soda

2 eggs, whisked

1 and ½ cups almond flour

¼ cup ghee, melted

1 tablespoon vanilla extract

1 cup blackberries, mashed

Cooking spray

Directions:

In a bowl, mix the flour with the baking powder, baking soda, stevia, vanilla and blackberries and stir well.

Add the rest of the ingredients, stir the batter and pour it into a loaf pan greased with cooking spray.

Bake at 400 degrees F for 1 hour, cool down, slice and serve.

Nutrition: calories 200, fat 7, fiber 3, carbs 5, protein 7

131. Keto Raspberries Bread

Preparation time: 10 minutes

Cooking time: 50 minutes

Servings: 6

Ingredients:

2 cups almond flour

1 teaspoon baking soda

¾ cup erythritol

A pinch of salt

1 egg

¾ cup coconut milk

¼ cup ghee, melted

2 cups raspberries

2 teaspoons vanilla extract

¼ cup coconut oil, melted

Directions:

In a bowl, mix the flour with the baking soda, erythritol, salt, vanilla and the raspberries and stir.

Add the rest of the ingredients gradually and mix the batter well.

Pour this into a lined loaf pan and bake at 350 degrees F for 50 minutes.

Cool the bread down, slice and serve.

Nutrition: calories 200, fat 7, fiber 3, carbs 5, protein 7

132. Simple Strawberry Bread

Preparation time: 10 minutes

Cooking time: 50 minutes

Servings: 8

Ingredients:

3 and ½ cups almond flour

2 cups strawberries, chopped

1 teaspoon baking soda

2 cups swerve

1 tablespoon cinnamon powder

4 eggs, whisked

1 and ¼ cups coconut oil, melted

Cooking spray

Directions:

In a bowl, mix the flour with baking soda, swerve, strawberries and the cinnamon and stir.

Add the remaining ingredients, stir the batter and pour this into 2 loaf pans greased with cooking spray.

Bake at 350 degrees F for 50 minutes, cool the bread down, slice and serve.

Nutrition: calories 221, fat 7, fiber 4, carbs 5, protein 3

133. Great Plum Bread

Preparation time: 10 minutes

Cooking time: 50 minutes

Servings: 8

Ingredients:

1 cup plums, pitted and chopped

1 and ½ cups coconut flour

¼ teaspoon baking soda

½ cup ghee, melted

A pinch of salt

1 and ¼ cups swerve

½ teaspoon vanilla extract

1/3 cup coconut cream

2 eggs, whisked

Directions:

In a bowl, mix the flour with baking soda, salt, swerve, and the vanilla and stir.

In a separate bowl, mix the plums with the remaining ingredients and stir.

Combine the 2 mixtures and stir the batter well.

Pour into 2 lined loaf pans and bake at 350 degrees F for 50 minutes.

Cool the bread down, slice and serve them.

Nutrition: calories 199, fat 8, fiber 3, carbs 6, protein 4

134. Lime Bread

Preparation time: 10 minutes

Cooking time: 50 minutes

Servings: 8

Ingredients:

2/3 cup ghee, melted

2 cups swerve

4 eggs, whisked

3 teaspoons baking powder

1 cup almond milk

2 tablespoons lime zest, grated

2 tablespoons lime juice

3 cups coconut flour

Cooking spray

Directions:

In a bowl, mix the flour with lime zest, baking powder and the swerve and stir.

In a separate bowl, mix the lime juice with the rest of the ingredients except the cooking spray and stir well.

Combine the 2 mixtures, stir the batter well and pour into 2 loaf pans greased with cooking spray and bake at 350 degrees F for 50 minutes.

Cool the bread down, slice and serve.

Nutrition: calories 203, fat 7, fiber 3, carbs 4, protein 6

135. Delicious Rhubarb Bread

Preparation time: 10 minutes

Cooking time: 40 minutes

Servings: 10

Ingredients:

1 cup almond milk

1 teaspoon vanilla extract

1 tablespoon lemon juice

2/3 cup coconut oil, melted

1 egg

1 and ½ cups swerve

2 an ½ cups coconut flour

A pinch of salt

2 cups rhubarb, chopped

1 teaspoon baking soda

½ teaspoon cinnamon powder

1 tablespoon ghee, melted

Cooking spray

Directions:

In a bowl, mix the vanilla with lemon juice, swerve, flour, salt, rhubarb, baking soda, and the cinnamon and stir.

Add the rest of the ingredients except the cooking spray, stir the batter and pour into a loaf pan greased with cooking spray.

Bake at 350 degrees F for 40 minutes, cool down, slice and serve.

Nutrition: calories 200, fat 7, fiber 2, carbs 4, protein 6

136. Delicious Cantaloupe Bread

Preparation time: 10 minutes

Cooking time: 1 hour

Servings: 8

Ingredients:

4 tablespoons stevia

3 eggs

1 cup coconut oil, melted

1 tablespoon vanilla extract

1 teaspoon baking powder

1 teaspoon baking soda

2 teaspoons cinnamon powder

½ teaspoon ginger, ground

2 cups cantaloupe, peeled and pureed

½ cup ghee, melted

3 cups almond flour

Directions:

In a bowl, mix the flour with ginger, cinnamon, baking soda, baking powder, vanilla and the stevia and stir.

Add the rest of the ingredients and stir the batter well.

Pour into 2 lined loaf pans and bake at 360 degrees F for 1 hour.

Cool the bread down, slice and serve.

Nutrition: calories 211, fat 8, fiber 3, carbs 6, protein 6

Thanks everyone!

Making bread can be so much fun! You can use so many different ingredients and flavors! The combinations are endless! The bread recipes collection you've just discovered shows you how to make the most delicious and textured ketogenic breads from the comfort of your own kitchen.

Anyone can enjoy these breads and you don't need to be an expert in the kitchen to make them. The Ketogenic breads gathered here are all so rich and delightful! Check out all of them and enjoy them!

Please continue reading for an awesome bonus...

Chapter 3. FREE FAT BOMB RECIPES BONUS!

137. Chocolate Peppermint Bombs

Ingredients
Servings: 19
Filling:

½ cup coconut oil

½ cup coconut butter

12 drops Stevia

1 tsp peppermint extract

Coating:

½ cup coconut oil

½ cup cacao powder

20 drops Stevia

1 tsp vanilla extract

Directions:

Melt the coconut oil and coconut butter together in a saucepan over a medium heat.

Transfer to a mixing bowl and add in the Stevia and peppermint extract. Mix well.

Spoon mixture into an ice cube tray or small cupcake liners. Use 2 tablespoons per mold. Freeze for 1 hour.

Meanwhile, mix together all the COATING ingredients in a mixing bowl. You will need to melt the coconut oil first.

Remove the now firm filling mixture from their mold and dip each one into the coating mixture. You can use a fork for this. Place on parchment paper and freeze when all are covered.

Serve when coating is solid!

Calories: 130 Carbs: 2g Fiber: 1g Fat: 13g Saturated Fat: 10g

138. 3 Ingredients Only Bombs

Ingredients
Servings: 12

1 cup almond butter

½ cup coconut flour

2 tablespoons Stevia

Directions:

Line a baking sheet with parchment paper.

Whisk together the butter, Stevia and coconut flour in a small bowl. Mix until thick, then allow to freeze for 15 minutes.

When 15 minutes is up, remove from freezer and roll into 12 small balls with your hands.

Place each ball onto the baking sheet then place back in freezer for 20 minutes until firm, then serve!

Calories: 75 Carbs: 1g Fat: 9g Saturated Fat: 4g Protein: 1.5g

139. Mocha Bombs

Ingredients
Servings: 12

1 cup cream cheese

4 tablespoons Swerve

2 tablespoons unsweetened cocoa

¼ cup coffee, chilled

½ cup dark chocolate, melted

1/8 cup cocoa butter, melted

Directions:

In a blender, mix together the coffee, cream cheese, cocoa and Swerve. Blend until smooth.

Roll out 12 small fat bombs from the mixture onto a plate lined with parchment paper.

Now mix together the melted dark chocolate and cocoa butter.

Roll each ball through the mixture in step 3 until fully covered. Place back on plate when all 12 are done.

Allow to set in freezer for 2 hours. Serve when ready!

Calories: 105 Carbs: 2.3g Fat: 12g Protein: 2g Fiber: 0.7g

140. Pumpkin Cheesecake Bombs

Ingredients
Servings: 14

8 ounces cream cheese

4 tablespoons Swerve

1/3 cup pumpkin puree

1 tsp pumpkin pie spice

1 tsp vanilla extract

2.5 tablespoons coconut flour

1/3 cup pecans, minced

1 tsp cinnamon

2 tablespoons Erythritol

Directions:

Line a baking sheet with parchment paper

With an electric mixer, beat together the cream cheese, swerve, pumpkin puree, pie spice, vanilla extract and coconut flour.

Place mixture and bowl in freezer for 15 minutes until the mixture is semi-firm. Meanwhile, combine the pecans, cinnamon and Erythritol in a separate bowl.

Remove mixture from freezer and form 14 small balls from it with your hands. Now roll each one into the pecan, cinnamon and Erythritol mixture until fully covered.

Re-freeze for 20 minutes then serve when desired!

Calories: 80 Carbs: 1.4g Fat: 9g Protein: 1.5g Fiber: 0.5g

141. Salted Caramel Peanut Butter bombs

Ingredients
Servings: 18

8 tablespoons butter, unsalted

1 cup coconut oil

1 cup natural chunky peanut butter

¼ cup sugar-free caramel syrup

Directions:

Over a medium heat, melt all the ingredients into a saucepan and mix thoroughly.

Pour mixture into ice-cube tray and place in the freezer for 1 hour or until visibly set.

Remove when firm and serve when desired!

Calories: 125 Carbs: 2.3g Fat: 22g Protein: 3g Fiber: 0.7g

142. Chocolate Coconut Almond Bombs

Ingredients
Servings: 30

½ cup coconut butter, melted

½ cup coconut oil, melted

1 tsp almond extract

¼ cup cocoa powder, unsweetened

½ tsp vanilla extract

10 drops Stevia

¼ cup almonds, crushed

¼ cup shredded coconut, unsweetened

¼ cup cacao nibs

Directions:

Melt the coconut butter and coconut oil over a medium heat in a saucepan. Then transfer it to a mixing bowl along with the cocoa powder, almond extract, vanilla extract and Stevia. Mix thoroughly.

Add the remaining ingredients and combine.

Fill mini cupcake liners with 1 tablespoon of mixture for each. This recipe should make around 3

Leave to firm in freezer for 30 minutes before serving.

Calories: 87 Carbs: 1g Fat: 7g Protein: 0.3g Fiber: 1g

143. Blackberry Fat Bombs

Ingredients
Servings: 16

1 cup coconut butter

1 cup coconut oil

½ tsp Stevia drops

½ cup frozen blackberries

½ tsp vanilla extract

1 tablespoon lemon juice

Directions:

Heat the coconut oil, coconut butter and frozen berries in a saucepan over a medium heat and stir until well combined.

Transfer the above mixture to a blender and add the remaining ingredients. Blend until smooth.

Pour the mixture out evenly into a pan lined with parchment paper. A 6x6 pan should be fine here.

Refrigerate for 1 hour. Remove when hardened and cut into 16 squares before serving!

Calories: 150 Carbs: 2.8g Fat: 17g Protein: 1g

144. Sea Salted Chocolate Bombs

Ingredients
Servings: 10

½ cup whipping cream

½ cup coconut oil

½ cup sunflower butter

1 tsp vanilla extract

2 tablespoons cocoa powder

1/3 cup cream cheese

1 tsp cinnamon

3 tablespoons grass-fed butter

2 tsp coarse sea salt

Directions:

In a medium sized bowl, whip the whipping cream until peaks form. Fold in the vanilla extract.

In a blender, mix together the remaining ingredients MINUS the sea salt. Blend until smooth.

Fold this mixture slowly into the whipping cream in step 1 and combine thoroughly.

Spoon mixture into silicone molds. This recipe should make around 10 fat bombs.

Sprinkle each with some sea salt then freeze for 6-8 hours before serving!

Calories: 102 Carbs: 2.8g Fat: 19g Protein: 1g

145. Vanilla Cheesecake Bombs

Ingredients
Servings: 16

8 ounces cream cheese

½ cup Splenda

1 cup heavy cream

2 tsp vanilla extract

Directions:

Add the cream cheese, Splenda and vanilla extract to a bowl and mix with a hand blender until smooth.

Add in the heavy cream and whisk until mixture is thick and produces firm peaks.

Spoon mixture into mini cupcake liners. If you can use a piping bag, then that's even better. This recipe should make around 16-20 fat bombs.

Set in fridge for 2 hours before serving!

Calories: 80 Carbs: 1g Fat: 10g Protein: 1g

146. Smooth and Crunchy Pecan Fat Bombs

Ingredients
Servings: 12

½ cup pecans

¼ cup ghee

¼ cup coconut butter

1/8 tsp salt

¼ cup coconut oil

½ tsp vanilla extract

Directions:

Toast the pecans in a skillet over a medium heat until darker. They should smell toasty when ready.

Now chop the pecans into reasonably large chunks. This comes down to personal preference, how big you have them.

In a different saucepan, melt the coconut butter, ghee and coconut oil together over a low heat. Now stir in the vanilla and salt.

Divide out the chopped pecans into the silicon mold of your choice. I prefer using a cubed mold that holds 12 for this recipe.

Pour the mixture over the pecans evenly then leave to freeze for 30 minutes until hard.

If you don't have a mold, you can simply freeze the mixture in a container then chop it up afterwards!

Calories: 142 Carbs: 2g Fat: 16g Saturated fat: 10g Fiber: 1g Protein: 1g

147. Key Lime Pie Bombs

Ingredients
Servings: 30

2 cups raw cashews

½ cup coconut butter

1 cup coconut oil

¾ cup key lime juice

¼ tsp Stevia

Directions:

Boil the cashew nuts for 12 minutes.

Melt the coconut oil over a medium heat in a saucepan.

Transfer the melted coconut oil to a food processor with all other ingredients, including cashews and blend until smooth.

Transfer mixture to a mixing bowl and leave in freezer for 30 minutes.

Form as many small balls as you can from the mixture. This recipe should make about 30 small fat bombs. Return these to the freezer for 20 minutes so they harden.

When ready to serve, leave them out to thaw a little beforehand.

Calories: 152 Carbs: 4g Fat: 15g Protein: 2g

148. Keto Mousse Bomb

Ingredients

Servings: 2

1 cup full fat mascarpone cheese

1 tablespoon Erythritol

1 tsp baking cocoa powder

Directions:

Simply mix together the mascarpone cheese, cocoa powder and Erythritol until mixture is smooth.

Leave in fridge for 10 mins before consuming!

Calories: 252 Carbs: 2g Fat: 25g Protein: 1.5g Fiber: 3.4g

149. Pumpkin Pie Fat Bombs

Ingredients
Servings: 12

½ cup shredded coconut, unsweetened

½ cup coconut oil

¼ cup collagen

20 drops Stevia

¼ tsp Himalayan salt

¾ cup pumpkin puree

1 tablespoon ground cinnamon

1 tsp ground ginger

¼ tsp vanilla extract

Pinch of ground cloves

Directions:

Line baking sheet with 12 mini muffin silicon molds.

In a blender, mix together the coconut oil, Stevia, shredded coconut and salt until smooth and drippy.

Remove a quarter cup of the above mixture, then add the remaining ingredients and blend again.

Pour this mixture evenly into the 12 molds. Press the mixture firmly into the mold.

Now, with the remaining quarter cup from step 3, pour this over the top of each fat bomb. This will create a layered effect.

Place on baking sheet then leave in freezer for 1 hour, then serve!

Calories: 202 Carbs: 2g Fat: 21g Protein: 3.5g Fiber: 3.4g

150. Pecan Peanut Crunch Fat Bombs

Ingredients
Servings: 16

2 cups chopped pecan nuts

4 tablespoons melted coconut oil

2 tablespoons melted grass-fed butter

2 tablespoon peanut butter (sugar-free if possible

2 tablespoon cocoa powder, unsweetened

½ tsp Stevia powder

Directions:

Melt the coconut oil and butter in a saucepan over medium heat, stirring well.

Finely chop the pecan nuts, then mix ALL the ingredients together in a medium-sized mixing bowl until fully combined.

Spoon the mixture into small cupcake molds, about 1 tablespoon per mold made me 16 fat bombs.

Leave in freezer for 15 minutes until firm.

Serve when desired. These can be stored in fridge or freezer.

Calories: 130 Carbs: 2.4g Fat: 15g Protein: 1.5g

151. Coffee Cheesecake Fat Bombs

Ingredients
Servings: 17

2 cups cream cheese

1 cup grass-fed butter

1/3 cup Stevia

2 tablespoons cocoa powder, unsweetened

3 tablespoons cold brew coffee

Directions:

Mix together the cream cheese, grass-fed butter and Stevia in a medium-sized bowl. Use a blender for best results.

Scoop out one cup of the above mixture and transfer it to a small bowl. Now add the cocoa powder to this mixture and stir until combined.

Add the cold coffee brew to the medium-sized bowl in step 1 and stir until combined.

For the best results, use a casserole dish of an 8"x8" size and line it with parchment paper.

Line the bottom of the casserole dish with the cocoa mixture from step This is your base, so to speak.

Now spread the other mixture over the top of this base, covering entirely.

Leave in freezer for 4 hours. Cut into squares when ready then serve.

Calories: 180 Carbs: 1.4g Fat: 20g Saturated Fat: 12g Protein: 1.5g

152. Ferrero Rocher Fat Bombs

Ingredients
Servings: 10

¾ cup ground hazelnuts

3 tablespoons coconut oil

2 tablespoons Erythritol

1 ounce dark chocolate (85% cocoa

½ tsp vanilla extract

½ tablespoon baking cocoa powder

½ cup chopped whole nuts and hazelnuts

Directions:

Melt the dark chocolate and coconut oil in a microwave or saucepan until fully melted.

Blend together the hazelnuts, Erythritol, cocoa powder and vanilla extract in a food processor. Now pour in the mixture from step 1 and blend again.

Place mixture in freezer for 10 minutes. Make 10 balls from the mixture with your hands by rolling each ball around a whole hazelnut so it sits in the middle of the mixture.

Roll each ball into the chopped whole nuts and hazelnuts until fully covered. Serve immediately!

Calories: 145 Carbs: 2.4g Fat: 14g Protein: 1.9g Fiber: 1.7g

153. Blueberry Fat Bombs

Ingredients
Servings: 12

¾ cup of cream cheese

½ cup blueberries

5 tablespoons butter

¼ tsp vanilla extract

3 tablespoons coconut oil

1/8 tsp sea salt

Directions:

Blend all the ingredients together in a food blender until smooth.

Spoon the mixture evenly into a parchment-lined loaf pan.

Freeze mixture for 1 hour until firm. Remove and cut into 12 pieces.

Return to freezer for another hour until mixture is solid. Remove from pan then serve!

Calories: 115 Carbs: 1g Fat: 12g Protein: 1g Fiber: 1.2g

154. Chocolate Tahini Fat Bombs

Ingredients
Servings: 16

2 ounces cacao butter

1 ounce cacao baking chocolate

¼ cup coconut oil

¼ cup Swerve

½ cup tahini

Flaky sea salt

Directions:

Melt together the coconut oil, baking chocolate and cacao butter in a small saucepan on a low heat. Stir while heating.

2.Whisk in the Swerve and tahini with the above mixture until fully combined.

Line a muffin tin with liners and scoop the mixture into each compartment.

Chill for 30 minutes before serving.

Calories: 125 Carbs: 1g Fat: 12g Protein:

155. Focaccia With Tomatoes And Rosemary

Servings: 6-8 slices
Preparation time: 45 mins
Cooking Time: 20 mins
Ingredients:
4 cups or 500g bread flour
1 tbsp. olive oil, plus extra to glaze
1⅓ cups or 320ml water
1 7g-sachet fast-action dried yeast
20 fresh cherry tomatoes, halved
2 sprigs fresh rosemary, leaves chopped
1½ tsp. salt
Coarse sea salt, for topping
Directions:
In a large mixing bowl, mix the flour, yeast and salt.
Pour in the olive oil and water. Stir with a large wooden spoon until the mixture has mostly come together into a dough.
Scrape the dough onto a clean work surface.
Knead the dough by holding one end in one hand and stretching it with the other hand.
Form the dough into a ball again, turn 90 degrees and start kneading again. Repeat for 10 minutes.
When the dough is smooth and shiny, put in a large mixing bowl, coat with a layer of olive oil and cover the bowl with a damp-dry kitchen towel.
Leave the dough in a warm, draft-free place for 1 – 2 hours, until the dough just about doubles in size.
Flatten the dough and shape into the traditional focaccia shape, then place in an oiled baking tin.
Poke deep holes into the focaccia (just above the bottom of the doughand push the cherry tomato halves (cut side facing upinto the focaccia.
 Coat the focaccia with olive oil and sprinkle with finely chopped rosemary and coarse salt.
 Preheat the oven to 480 degrees Fahrenheit.
 Cover with a damp-dry kitchen towel and prove in the tin for another 30 minutes.
 Bake for 10 minutes and then turn the oven down to 390 degrees Fahrenheit and bake another 10-15 minutes until the top is a light golden brown.

156. Vegan Pide Bread

Servings: 1 loaf

Preparation time: 15 mins

Cooking Time: 15 mins

Ingredients:

2 cups all-purpose flour

1 tsp. white sesame seeds

1 tsp. black sesame seeds

½ cup water

1 tbsp. olive oil

1 tsp. instant yeast

1 tsp. olive oil

1 pinch sugar

½ tsp. salt

Directions:

Put all the recipe ingredients in the bowl of a stand mixer to make a dough. You may also mix by hand but it's easier done with a stand mixer.

Prove until the dough just about doubles in size.

Pre-heat the oven to 500 degrees Fahrenheit.

Place the dough onto a lightly oiled baking tray and flatten the dough with your hands.

Add 1 teaspoon olive oil and sprinkle on the sesame seeds. Work these toppings into the dough while spreading all over.

Bake for about 15 minutes or until the bread begins to go a light golden brown.

Nutrition:

Total Calories: 1134 kcal. Calories from Fat: 207 kcal.

Total Carbohydrates 197g (Dietary Fiber 9g, Sugars 1g), Protein 31g, Total Fat 23g (Saturated Fat 3g), Sodium 1180mg, Potassium 382mg.

157. Garlic-Herb Flatbread

Servings: 6 flatbreads

Preparation time: 1 hr. 30 mins

Cooking Time: 30 mins

Ingredients:

1¼ cups unbleached all-purpose flour

¾ cup spelt flour 1 packet or 2¼ tsp. active dry yeast

1 tbsp. olive oil, plus extra for coating

¾ cup warm water

2 cloves or 1 tbsp. fresh garlic, minced

½ tsp. organic cane sugar

½ tbsp. fresh thyme, finely chopped

½ tbsp. fresh rosemary, finely chopped

¾ tsp. sea salt

Directions:

Add yeast, herbs, garlic, organic cane sugar, sea salt, all-purpose flour, and spelt flour. Stir well.

Create space in the dry ingredients and add the olive oil, adding ½ cup of the warm water to start. Stir with a wooden spoon, adding more water until a dough forms.

Scrape the dough onto a well-floured surface and knead for 2 minutes until elastic and smooth. Slowly add more flour to prevent sticking.

Using kitchen paper, wipe the bowl and lightly coat. Roll the dough around in the bowl to coat and cover with a clean damp-dry kitchen towel or cling film. Prove in a warm, draft-free place for 1 hour.

Divide the dough into 6 even portions and arrange on a clean lightly floured worktop. Cover with a clean damp-dry kitchen towel and rest.

Heat a large cast iron skillet in a 375-degree-Fahrenheit oven to a medium-high heat

Roll each dough piece into a large fairly thin circle about a ⅛ of an inch thick.

Lightly oil the preheated cast iron skillet and lay the flatbread on it.

Cook untouched for 2½ minutes and then flip over and cook for 2½ minutes on the second side.

Repeat, adding more oil to the skillet, until all the flatbreads are cooked.

Enjoy immediately!

  You may also cool the flatbreads and store in a well-sealed Ziploc bag or airtight container up to 3 days. However, these flatbreads are best eaten fresh.

Nutrition:

Total Calories: 175 kcal.

Total Carbohydrates: 32.6g (Dietary Fiber: 3g Sugar: 0.8g), Protein: 5.3g, Fat: 3g, Sodium: 270mg.

158. Yeast-Free Flatbread

Servings: 8 flatbreads

Preparation time: 20 mins

Cooking Time: 5 mins

Ingredients:

2 cups unbleached all-purpose flour, plus extra for rolling and flouring

½ cup water

¼ cup almond milk (making the recipe dairy-free

2 tbsp. olive oil

1 tbsp. baking powder

½ tsp. salt

Directions:

Combine all of the ingredients in a food processor, using a dough blade or a stand-mixer with a dough hook attachment. Process until a dough ball forms.

You may also mix by hand and stir until the dough comes out soft and pliable but not sticky.

Scrape the dough onto a clean floured surface and divide the dough in half. Roll into smooth dough balls.

From these 2 dough balls create 8 equal dough portions.

Line a baking sheet with baking parchment paper.

Take one dough ball and flatten into a rough circle.

Using a rolling pin, roll out a 5 to 6-inch circle.

Place the flat dough onto the prepared baking sheet and repeat until you have 3 flat dough circles.

Cover with baking parchment and continue rolling the remaining 4 dough balls, laying them onto the baking parchment.

Heat a griddle over a medium-high heat.

Place one of the dough circles and cook until bubbles begin forming and the edges begin to lift. This takes 1 to 2 minutes.

Quickly flip over the flatbread and cook for 1 - 2 minutes.

Remove from the griddle and place onto a clean, dry plate. Keep warm by covering with a dry kitchen towel. Repeat until all flatbreads are cooked.

Serve immediately!

These flatbreads can be stored an airtight container or in the fridge for 3 - 4 days.

159. Navajo Flatbread

Servings: 10 flatbreads

Preparation time: 15 mins

Cooking Time: 10 mins

Ingredients:

600g strong white bread flour, plus more for rolling and dusting

6 tbsp. olive oil

2 tbsp. baking powder

150ml warm water

1 tsp. fine sea salt

1 tsp. dried herbs, such as parsley, chili, thyme, crushed fennel seeds, cumin or sumac (optional

Directions:

Mix the flour, herbs or spices (if using), salt and baking powder in a large bowl.

Clear a well in the center of the flour, then pour in the olive oil and about 150ml of warm water.

Using a fork slowly center in the flour from the edges of the bowl, adding in water if you think the dough is too dry.

Once the dough begins to combine, wet your hands and use to form the dough into a nice ball of dough.

Flour your hands and scrape the dough onto a clean work surface.

Knead the dough until smooth and elastic. This should take between 5 - 10 minutes.

Place the dough back into the bowl, dust with more flour, then cover.

Divide the dough into 10 equal dough ball portions, and with lightly oiled hands, squeeze each ball between your palms flattening slightly.

Dust with flour as you go, patting and slapping the dough from one hand to the other.

Keep turning and twisting the dough in a circular movement and keep throwing the dough from hand to hand, until each flatbread is about 1cm thick.

Cooking flatbreads is usually a continuous process. As you make some, simultaneously cook others, keeping an eye on them to prevent overcooking or burning.

Cook on the stovetop in a non-stick pan or on the barbeque, on a medium heat.

Cook for a 1 - 2 minutes on each side, checking the underside. The flatbreads should puff up and develop a light golden color.

Place in a food basket or plate covered with clean, dry kitchen towel, until they're ready to be served.

Serve warm with anything from salads, curries, stews, soups or even burgers!

Nutrition:

Total Calories: 271 kcal.

Total Carbohydrates 42.5g (Sugars 0.8g), Fat 7.4g (Saturated Fat 1.1g), Protein 7.8g.

160. Spelt Chapatti

Servings: 2 flatbreads

Preparation time: 10 mins

Cooking Time: 5 mins

Ingredients:

⅓ cup spelt flour

2 tbsp. lukewarm water

¼ tsp. salt, plus more to sprinkle

½ tsp. white sesame seeds (optional

Directions:

In a large mixing bowl, combine the spelt flour and salt and mix.

Slowly add water, a little at a time until a smooth dough is formed. You might not need all of the water, keep an eye on the addition of the water to keep from forming a wet dough.

Knead the dough until smooth. You may also use a stand mixer with a dough hook attachment, but for this small amount of ingredients, it is perfectly fine to use your hands.

Rest the dough in a bowl covered with a clean, dry kitchen towel for about 30 minutes.

Divide the dough equally in two and roll out into chapattis on a floured surface.

You may sprinkle sesame seeds and additional salt over the flatbreads, rolling the seeds and salt into the dough.

Heat a non-stick crepe pan or any other flat pan you may have, and try to get it as hot as you possibly can.

Place 1 chapatti in the hot crepe pan and cook for about 30 seconds on each side, moving them constantly so that they don't burn.

Place on a plate and cover with the dry kitchen towel while you cook the second chapatti.

 Serve immediately with the veggie curry of your choice and enjoy!

Nutrition:

Total Calories 82 kcal.

Total Carbohydrates 14g (Dietary Fiber 2g), Protein 2g, Sodium 292mg.

161. Wholemeal Chapatti

Servings: 8 chapattis

Preparation time: 30 mins

Cooking Time: 10 mins

Ingredients:

1 lb. or 450g whole meal chapatti flour (substitute with whole meal plain flour

9 fl. oz. or 200 ml cold water

1 tsp. salt

Butter or ghee for spreading (optional

Directions:

Set aside 7 oz. or 200g of the flour and reserve for rolling the chapattis, and then put the remaining flour and salt in a large bowl.

Fill a mixing jug with the cold water.

Add water to the bowl of flour, little by little, as you knead, until you have a smooth, soft, and elastic dough. The longer you knead the softer the chapattis.

Sprinkle some of the reserved flour onto a clean work surface.

Divide the dough into eight portions and shape each portion into a ball.

Flatten the balls and then place one onto the floured work surface.

Roll out a flat disc of approximately 6 inches or 15cm in diameter, flouring as you go to form the chapattis.

Heat a griddle or a flat non-stick pan and get it as hot as you can.

Place each chapatti on the pan, or if using the griddle and cook for 20-30 seconds, until the surface begins to bubble.

 Flip over and cook on the other side for 10-15 seconds. Look out for brown spots, and as soon as they appear on the underside, remove the chapatti, it's done.

 Repeat with the remaining chapatti dough, using the remaining flour to roll.

 Stack up the chapattis as they cook, placing a sheet of kitchen paper between each piece to absorb any moisture.

 You may spread butter or ghee over one side, if you desire.

 Serve warm.

162. Pita Bread

Servings: 10 pita breads

Preparation time: 1 hr.

Cooking Time: 30 mins

Ingredients:

1 cup unbleached white flour or all-purpose flour

½ cup wheat flour

¾ cup warm water

1 tbsp. oil

¼ tsp. sugar

½ tsp. active yeast

⅓ tsp. salt

Extra wheat flour, for rolling and dusting

Directions:

Mix the yeast, sugar and warm water and rest for 2 minutes.

Then mix in salt into the white and whole wheat flours and add to the bowl containing the yeast mixture.

Add in the oil and knead until a soft dough forms about 1 – 2 minutes. Be careful not to over knead.

Cover with a clean, dry kitchen towel and prove for 1 hour in a warm, draft-free place until just about doubled in size.

Punch the dough down, flour it and knead for a few seconds to smooth.

Divide the dough into 10 equal portions. Roll each of the balls out in to 5 - 6 inch circles. Cover with the kitchen towel.

If cooking on the stove top, heat a cast iron skillet over a medium high heat.

Cook the pitta for 1 - 2 minutes or until the dough begins to bubble. Flip over and cook for another 30 seconds to 1 minute.

Then place the pitta on to the open flame. Keep the pita moving, flipping it over every few seconds until it is quite golden and puffed up.

 If baking in the oven, preheat to 450 degrees Fahrenheit.

 Place a large baking sheet or pizza stone in the oven to heat up for 20 minutes.

 Place the rolled pitas, 3 to 4 at a time, depending on the size of the baking sheet or stone.

Bake for 3 - 6 minutes, until the pitas puff up and develop a light golden color.

Switch the oven to a high broil setting and briefly broil the pita breads.

Once done, remove them carefully and bake the next batch.

Store the pita breads wrapped in a clean, dry kitchen towel for the day or in the fridge for up to 5 days.

Nutrition:

Total Calories 83 kcal. Calories from Fat: 9 kcal.

Total Carbohydrates 14g, Protein 2g, Total Fat 1g, Sodium 78mg, Potassium 20mg.

163. Pizza Dough

Servings: 10 slices

Preparation time: 10 mins

Cooking Time: 30 mins

Ingredients:

3 - 3½ cups flour

1 cup very warm water, at a temperature of 110-115F

2 tbsp. olive oil

2½ oz. fast rising yeast

1 tsp. salt

Directions:

Preheat the oven to 400 degrees Fahrenheit.

Combine flour, yeast, and salt in a large mixing bowl.

Add in the olive oil and warm water, and then knead for about 5 minutes or until the mixture is well combined. A smooth dough should form.

Rest the dough for 10 minutes in a warm, draft-free place.

Then roll out the dough until it fits on an oiled baking sheet, pizza stone or pizza pan.

Bake for approximately 10 minutes or until the crust is very slightly browned.

Remove from oven and cool.

Add the pizza toppings of your choice. You may use marinara, mozzarella, basil, prosciutto and mushrooms.

Return the pizza to oven and bake for 10-20 minutes or until all the cheese is melted.

 Cool, slice, and serve.

164. Cauliflower Pizza Crust

Servings: 2

Preparation time: 20 mins

Cooking Time: 30 mins

Ingredients:

1 lb. cauliflower florets (fresh or frozen

½ cup almond meal

3 tbsp. ground chia or flax seeds, divided into 2 portions

3 - 6 tbsp. water, as needed

½ tsp. dried oregano

½ tsp. garlic powder

½ tsp. salt

Directions:

Line a baking sheet with baking parchment paper.

Preheat the oven to 400 degrees Fahrenheit.

Place the cauliflower florets in the bowl of a food processor fitted with an S blade.

Pulse until the cauliflower forms a rice-like texture.

Pour the cauliflower "rice" into a large sauce pan, add enough water to cover, and heat until boiling.

Cover, lower the heat, and allow to the cauliflower rice to simmer for 5 minutes.

Drain the liquid, transfer the cooked cauliflower rice into a freezer-safe bowl and freeze for 10 minutes.

Mix 2 tablespoons of ground chia or flax seeds with 3 tablespoons of water, and allow to gel forming a vegan "egg." Set aside.

Remove the cooled cauliflower rice from the freezer and pour onto the center of a thin dry kitchen towel.

Squeeze the rice, removing all excess water.

Place the drained cauliflower into a bowl, and then tip in the vegan "egg" mixture, an additional tablespoon a ground flax or chia seeds, almond meal, garlic, dried oregano and salt.

Add 3 more tablespoons of water, only if you fell the dough needs it, and stir.

Press the cauliflower "dough" until ¼ inch thick and spread to fill the baking-parchment-lined baking sheet. Make sure that there are no "thin spots" as the dough might crack.

Bake at 400 degrees Fahrenheit for 30 minutes, until the top is a light golden color and dry to touch.

For the best texture, use an additional piece of baking parchment paper to flip the entire crust, and then return to the sheet pan. Bake for a further 15 minutes.

Once the crust is firm, add your favorite vegan toppings (like onions, fresh spinach, marinara or cashew parmesanand bake briefly about 5-10 additional minutes.

Recipe Notes:

If using frozen cauliflower, you can skip the cooking and cooling process. Thaw the frozen cauliflower overnight, and then pulse the thawed cauliflower to form the rice. Squeeze and drain excess water using a dry tea towel.

165. Flour Tortillas

Servings: 4 tortillas

Preparation time: 12 mins

Cooking Time: 8 mins

Ingredients:

1 cup whole grain flour

2 tbsp. olive oil

¼ cup water

⅛ tsp. salt

Extra flour, for rolling and flouring

Directions:

Mix all the ingredients in a bowl and using a spoon or fork form into a smooth dough. If it comes out too dry, add a little more water.

Divide the dough into 4 equal portions. Flour a flat surface and place the dough ball on it.

Press down onto the ball until the dough is fairly flat. Keep flouring both your hands and the work surface to stop the dough from sticking.

Use a rolling pin or to flatten the dough into a thin circle. Keep flattening the dough, flouring both it and the dough circle, spinning it as you go along.

Flash cook the tortillas on a high heat. Heat up a large flat pan on the stove top. When the pan is hot enough, place in the first tortilla.

Cook for 30 seconds per side until brown spots begin to appear.

When both sides are done, take the tortilla out place onto a plate. Repeat the process until all the tortillas are cooked

Enjoy immediately!

Nutrition:

Total Calories: 190 kcal. Calories from Fat: 72 kcal.

Total Carbohydrates 26g (Dietary Fiber 4g, Protein 5g), Total Fat 8g (Saturated Fat 1g), Sodium 78mg, Potassium 130mg

166. Afghan Naan

Servings: 2 naan

Preparation time: 2 hrs. 30 mins

Cooking Time: 10 mins

Ingredients:

3 cups bread flour, plus 1 tablespoon more

1 cup warm water

1 packet quick-acting yeast

2 tsp. oil

1 tsp. sugar

1 tsp. salt

Extra warm water, for kneading

Vegan butter, for brushing (optional

Nigella seeds (optional

Directions:

Mix the yeast, sugar and warm water, and leave to sponge for 10 minutes. The mixture will look foamy when ready.

Combine the flour, oil and salt, in large a mixing bowl.

Pour the yeast mixture into the bowl with the flour and mix using a wooden spoon, until the dough is just about to form.

At this stage, use your hands to knead the dough for 5 minutes.

Cover with a clean, dry towel or cling film and prove in a warm place for 1-2 hours.

Punch down the dough to remove the air within and divide the dough into 2 equal portions.

Preheat the oven to 400 degrees Fahrenheit.

Combine 5 tablespoons water with the extra 1 tablespoon of flour and mix well to make a liquid mixture free of any lumps.

Apply some of the flour mixture to your hands and then flatten the dough ball into the traditional naan oval shape 10 – 12 inches long and 1/3 inch thick.

 Draw patterns into the dough with a fork and sprinkle n nigella seeds.

 Bake for 8-10 minutes, or until a light golden brown.

 The naan is now ready. You may also broil the naan for 2 minutes to completely brown the tops, but this is not very necessary.

Apply the vegan butter onto the naan, wrap them in a dry, clean kitchen towel to keep them soft and warm until ready to serve.

Enjoy a curry!

167. Sweet Potato Flatbread

Servings: 5 servings

Preparation time: 30 mins

Cooking Time: 3 mins

Ingredients:

For the Potato Puree:

1 medium sweet potato

1½ cup water

For the Dough:

1 cup sweet potato puree

1 cup tapioca flour

1 cup gluten-free flour blend

1 tsp. baking powder

For the Sweet version:

2 tbsp. coconut sugar

1 tsp. cinnamon

For the Savory version:

1 tsp. salt

Directions:

Peel and chop the sweet potato.

Boil in a medium saucepan, until tender. Once cooked, do not drain.

Puree the potato together with its cooking water in a blender until smooth.

Transfer to a bowl and immediately wash your blender.

Combine all the dry ingredients in a medium mixing bowl, and add 1 cup of the potato puree.

Knead everything to form a slightly sticky dough. Adjust for stickiness by adding ¼ cup more gluten-free flour.

Divide the dough into 5 equal portions.

Roll out each dough ball between two wax paper pieces to about 1-cm thickness.

Heat a non-stick skillet on a medium-high heat and place one flatbread into the pan. Cook for 1 to 1½ minutes or until the dough begins to bubble.

 Flip over and cook for another 1 to 1½ minutes on the other side. There should be brown spots on each side.

Remove from the heat and place in on a plate under a damp-dry kitchen towel to keep flatbreads soft while cooking the others.

Serve warm.

These flatbreads keep well in airtight container and refrigerated for up to 4 days. Reheat as above.

Chapter 4. Holiday Bread

168. Squash Muffins

Servings: 6

Nutrition:

3.4 g Net Carbs; 7.3 g Proteins; 7.8 g Fat; 111 Calories

Ingredients:

Salt – to taste

Baking powder - .66 tsp.

Almond flour – 1 cup

Peeled & grated squash – 1

Chopped spring onions – 2-3 sprigs

Olive oil – 1 tbsp.

Egg – 1

Plain yogurt - .25 cup

Grated hard cheese - .5 cup

Directions:

Warm up the oven to 350ºF. Spritz six muffin tins with cooking oil spray.

Season the grated squash with salt and set aside.

Combine the baking powder, salt, and sifted flour.

Whisk the egg, and mix with the oil, 1/2 of the cheese, and yogurt. Combine the fixings.

Add the squash and juices to the dough. Work in the chopped onions and add to the prepared muffin cups (1/2 full). Sprinkle with the cheese and bake for 25 minutes.

Cool slightly and serve. Store in the fridge when cooled if you have leftovers.

169. Zucchini Bread – Slow-Cooked

Servings: 12

Nutrition:

13.8 g Net Carbs ; 5 g Proteins; 15.7 g Fat; 174 Calories

Ingredients:

Cinnamon - 2 tsp.

Almond flour – 1 cup

Coconut flour - .33 cup

Optional: Xanthan gum - .5 tsp.

Salt - .5 tsp.

Baking soda - .5 tsp.

Baking powder – 1.5 tsp.

Softened coconut oil/butter - .33 cup

Eggs - 3

Vanilla – 2 tsp.

Sweetener – 1 cup or Pyure all-purpose - .5 cup

Shredded zucchini – 2 cups

Chopped pecans/walnuts - .5 cup

Also Needed: 8 x 4 silicone bread

pan

Directions:

Combine the coconut and almond flour, salt, baking soda and powder, xanthan gum, and cinnamon. Set aside for now.

Mix the oil, eggs, vanilla, and sugar in another dish. Combine the fixings.

Blend in the nuts and shredded zucchini. Scoop the mixture into the prepared bread pan.

Arrange the cooker on the top rack (or on crunched up aluminum foil balls). You want it at least 1/2-inch from the bottom of the slow cooker.

Secure the top tightly, and cook for three hours on the high setting.

Cool and wrap the bread in a sheet of foil. It's best when refrigerated.

170. Biscuits & Gravy

Servings: 8

Nutrition:

5 g Net Carbs; 17.4 g Proteins; 40 g Fat; 460 Calories

Ingredients for the Biscuits:

Baking powder – 1 tsp.

Almond flour – 1 cup

Celtic sea salt - .25 tsp.

Egg white - 4

Organic butter/cold coconut oil – 2 tbsp.

Optional: Garlic or another preferred spice – 1 tsp.

Ingredients for the Gravy:

Chicken/beef broth – 1 cup

Cream cheese – 1 cup

Ground black pepper – 1 pinch

Celtic sea salt – to your liking

Organic crumbled pork sausage - 1 pkg. (10 oz.

Also Needed: Coconut oil cooking spray

Directions:

Program the oven setting to 400ºF. Prepare a muffin pan/cookie sheet with the cooking spray.

Cut the butter up into pieces – making sure they are cold. Whisk the whites until fluffy.

In another container, combine the flour and baking powder. Cut in the butter and add the salt. Fold in the mixture over the egg whites.

Drop the dough onto the baking pan/muffin tin. Bake 11-15 minutes.

171. Buttery Garlic & Sharp Cheddar Biscuits

Servings: 8

Nutrition:

0.5 g Net Carbs; 6.7 g Proteins; 12.8 g Fat; 144 Calories

Ingredients:

Eggs - 4

Melted – slightly cooled – butter - .25 cup

Baking powder - .25 tsp.

Sifted coconut flour - .33 cup

Salt - .25 tsp.

Garlic powder - .25 tsp.

Shredded sharp cheddar cheese - 1 cup

Directions:

Set the oven temperature to 400ºF. Cover a baking tin with a sheet of aluminum foil. Grease with a spritz of oil.

Whisk the garlic powder, butter, eggs, and salt together. Fold in the baking powder and flour. Whisk until the lumps are removed. Stir in the cheese, mixing well.

Drop by the ice cream scoopful onto the baking pan. Bake about 15 min. Cool. Remove and serve.

They will lose the crispy texture if you don't cool first before you add them to a storage container.

172. Cheddar Bay Biscuits

Servings: 4 - 8 biscuits – 2 per serving

Nutrition: 2 g Net Carbs ;20 g Fat; 13 g Protein; 230 Calories

Ingredients:

Shredded mozzarella cheese – 1.5 cups

Shredded cheddar cheese – 1 cup

Cream cheese – .5 of 1 pkg. - 4 oz.

Large eggs – 2

Almond flour - .66 cup

Granulated garlic powder - .5 tsp.

Baking powder - 4 tsp.

Butter – for the pan

Directions:

Microwave for about 45 seconds using the high-power setting until melted. Stir and return for 20 additional seconds. Stir once more.

In another container, combine the eggs with the almond flour, garlic powder, and baking powder. Mix it all together and place on a sheet of flour-dusted plastic wrap. Roll and place in the fridge for 20-30 minutes.

Heat up the oven to reach 425ºF. Prepare a dark color baking dish with butter. Slice the cold dough into eight segments. Place in the prepared pan – leaving a little space between each one.

Bake for 10-12 minutes. Remove and place on the countertop to cool.

173. Lavender Biscuits

Servings: 6

Nutrition: 4 g Net Carbs; 10 g Proteins; 25 g Fat; 270 Calories

Ingredients:

Coconut oil - .33 cup

Baking powder – 1 tsp.

Almond flour – 1.5 cups

Kosher salt – 1 pinch

Egg whites - 4

Culinary grade lavender buds – 1 tbsp.

Liquid stevia – 4 drops

Directions:

Warm up the oven until it reaches 350ºF. Spritz a baking sheet with a little coconut oil. Mix the coconut oil and almond flour in a container until it's in pea-sized pieces. (It's easier to use your hands.Set the bowl aside in the fridge.

Whisk the eggs until they start foaming. Toss in the salt, lavender, and baking powder. Stir well and mix in the eggs. Add to the almond mixture, stirring well.

Place the chunks onto the baking sheet using an ice cream scoop or tablespoon. Pat them, so they aren't round similar to a pancake.

Bake for 20 minutes and enjoy.

Intermediate

174. Almond & Flax Crackers

Servings:20-24 crackers

Nutrition: Calories: 47.7, Total Fat: 5.2 g, Saturated Fat: 1 g, Carbs: 1.2 g, Sugars: 0.1 g, Protein: 1.9 g

Ingredients:

½ cup Ground Flax Seeds

½ cup Almond Flour

1 Tbsp Coconut Flour

2 Tbsp Shelled Hemp Seeds

¼ tsp Fine Sea Salt

1 Egg White

2 Tbsp Unsalted Butter, melted

Directions:

Preheat your oven to 300F / 150C.

Combine the flax, almond, and coconut flour, hemp seed, and salt. Add the egg and melted butter and mix until well combined.

Transfer the dough onto a sheet of parchment paper, cover with another sheet of paper and roll out the dough. Cut into crackers and arrange them on the prepared baking sheet.

Bake for half an hour, allow to cool and serve.

175. Chili Crackers

Servings: 30 crackers

Nutrition: Calories: 49, Total Fat: 4.1 g, Saturated Fat: 1.2 g, Carbs: 2.8 g, Sugars: 0.1 g, Protein: 1.6 g

Ingredients:

¾ cup Almond Flour

¼ cup Coconut Flour

¼ cup Flax Seed

½ tsp Paprika

½ tsp Cumin

1 1/2 tsp Chili Pepper Spice

1 tsp Onion Powder

½ tsp Salt

1 Egg

¼ cup Unsalted Butter

Directions:

Preheat your oven to 350F / 175C.

Pulse the ingredients until dough forms.

Divide the dough into two equal parts. Cut into crackers and repeat the same with the other ball of dough. Transfer the crackers to the prepared baking tray.

Bake for about 8-10 minutes. When done, remove from the oven, leave to cool and serve.

176. Cauliflower Gratin

All out: 50 min

Prep: 20 min

Cook: 30 min

Servings: 4 to 6

Ingredients

1 (3-poundhead cauliflower, cut into enormous florets

Fit salt

4 tablespoons (1/2 stickunsalted margarine, partitioned

3 tablespoons universally handy flour

2 cups hot milk

1/2 teaspoon naturally ground dark pepper

1/4 teaspoon ground nutmeg

3/4 cup naturally ground Gruyere, partitioned

1/2 cup naturally ground Parmesan

1/4 cup crisp bread scraps

Direction

Preheat the broiler to 375 degrees F.

Cook the cauliflower florets in an enormous pot of bubbling salted water for 5 to 6 minutes, until delicate yet at the same time firm. Channel.

In the mean time, liquefy 2 tablespoons of the spread in a medium pot over low warmth. Include the flour, mixing continually with a wooden spoon for 2 minutes. Empty the hot milk into the spread flour blend and mix until it reaches boiling point. Bubble, whisking continually, for 1 minute, or until thickened. Off the warmth, include 1 teaspoon of salt, the pepper, nutmeg, 1/2 cup of the Gruyere, and the Parmesan.

Pour 1/3 of the sauce on the base of a 8 by 11 by 2-inch preparing dish. Spot the depleted cauliflower on top and after that spread the remainder of the sauce uniformly on top. Consolidate the bread pieces with the rest of the 1/4 cup of Gruyere and sprinkle on top. Soften the rest of the 2 tablespoons of margarine and sprinkle over the gratin. Sprinkle with salt and pepper. Prepare for 25 to 30 minutes, until the top is sautéed. Serve hot or at room temperature.

177. Prosciutto, Rosemary And Pepper Bread

Servings: 1 huge portion, around 12 serving

Ingredients

1 bundle (2 1/2 teaspoonsdynamic dry yeast

1/4 cup warm (105 to 110 degrees Fwater

2 tablespoons additional virgin olive oil

1/2 teaspoons salt

3/4 teaspoon coarsely broke dark pepper

3 1/2 cups bread or unbleached generally useful flour, around

4 ounces (1/4-inch thickcut prosciutto, hacked into 1/4-inch dice

1/2 tablespoons slashed crisp rosemary or 2 teaspoons dried rosemary

Direction

In an enormous bowl or in the bowl of a rock solid electric blender, sprinkle the yeast over the water and mix. Let remain until the yeast mellow, around 10 minutes. Mix to break up the yeast.

Utilizing a wooden spoon or the oar sharp edge of the blender, mix in the oil, salt and pepper. Slowly beat in enough flour to make a shaggy mixture that clears the sides of the bowl.

In the case of manipulating by hand, turn out the batter onto a daintily floured work surface. Manipulate the batter, including more flour as required, until the mixture is smooth and versatile, around 10 minutes.

In the case of working by machine, change to the batter snare and manipulate on medium-low speed until the mixture is smooth and flexible, around 8 minutes. Whenever wanted, manipulate on the work surface to check the consistency.

Shape the mixture into a ball. Move the batter to a delicately oiled enormous bowl. Go to coat the mixture with oil. Spread firmly with saran wrap. Give stand access a warm spot until multiplied in volume, around 60 minutes.

Punch down the mixture and shape into a ball. Return the batter to the bowl, go to coat with oil, spread and let ascend until multiplied once more, around 45 minutes.

Position a rack in the focal point of the stove and preheat to 400 degrees F. Softly oil a huge preparing sheet.

Turn out the batter onto the work surface. Ply, continuously working in the prosciutto and rosemary. Smooth the batter into a 12-inch circle. Beginning at a long end, move up jam move style. Squeeze the creases shut. Spot on a preparing sheet, crease side down. Spread freely with saran wrap. Let ascend until multiplied in volume, around 30 minutes.

Utilizing a sharp blade, cut 3 shallow inclining cuts in the highest point of the bread. Prepare until the bread is brilliant darker and sounds empty when tapped on the last, 35 to 40 minutes. Cool totally on a wire rack. Whenever wanted, enclose by aluminum foil and store at room temperature as long as 8 hours before serving.

178. Keto Mousse Cake

Preparation Time: 1 hour

Servings:8

Nutrition:

Fat: 38 g.

Protein: 8 g.

Carbs: 10 g.

Ingredients:

For the Crust

1.5 cups Almond Flour

¼ cup Unsweetened Cocoa Powder

¼ cup Erythritol

½ cup Melted Butter

For the Filling

1.5 cups Cream Cheese

½ cup Dark Chocolate Chips, melted

½ cup Erythritol

1 tsp Vanilla Extract

1 tbsp Gelatin

1 cup Boiling Water

Directions:

All ingredients should be combined for the crust in a bowl. Mix well. Pack the mixture into a 9-inch springform pan.

Combine gelatin and erythritol in a bowl. Stir in a cup of boiling water. Leave for 5 minutes.

Beat cream cheese, melted chocolate, and vanilla in a separate bowl until light and airy.

Gradually stir in the gelatin mixture into the cream cheese mixture. Chill the mixture for 30 minutes then spread onto the crust.

Set the prepared cake in the chiller until ready to serve.

179. Jalapeno Cornbread Mini-Loaves

Servings: 8

Nutrition:

2.96 g Net Carbs; 11.2 g Proteins; 26.8 g Fat; 302 Calories

Ingredients for the Dry Ingredients:

Almond flour – 1.5 cups

Golden flaxseed meal - .5 cup

Salt – 1 tsp.

Baking powder – 2 tsp.

Ingredients for the Wet Ingredients:

Full fat sour cream - .5 cup

Melted butter – 4 tbsp.

Large eggs - 4

Liquid stevia – 10 drops

Amoretti sweet corn extract – 1 tsp.

Ingredients for the Add-Ins:

Grated sharp cheddar cheese - .5 cup

Fresh jalapenos, seeded

and membranes removed - 2

Directions:

Warm up the oven to reach 375ºF.

Spritz each of the loaf pans with oil cooking spray or butter.

Whisk or sift the dry fixings (salt, baking powder, almond flour, and flaxseed meal).

In another container, whisk the wet fixings and combine. Fold in the grated cheese and peppers. Pour into the pans and top off each one with a pepper ring.

Bake until golden brown or about 20-22 minutes. Leave it in the pan for about five minutes to cool. Then, just place on a wire rack before storing or serving.

Expert

180. Microwave Bread

Serving Size: 4 small rounds

Nutrition: 2 g Net Carbs; 3.25 g Proteins; 13 g Fat;132 Calories

Ingredients:

Almond flour - .33 cup

Salt - .125 tsp

Baking powder - .5 tsp

Melted ghee – 2.5 tbsp.

Whisked egg – 1

Oil – spritz for the mug

Directions:

Grease a cup with the oil. Combine all of the fixings in a mixing dish and pour into the cup. Put the cup in the microwave. Set the timer using the high setting for 90 seconds.

Transfer the mug to a cooling space for 2-3 minutes. Gently remove from the bread and slice into 4 portions.

181. Paleo Bread – Keto Style

Servings: 1 loaf – 10 slices

Nutrition: 9.1 g Net Carbs ; 10.4 g Proteins; 58.7 g Fat; 579.6 Calories

Ingredients:

Olive oil - .5 cup (+2 tbsp.

Eggs – 3

Almond milk/water - .25 cup

Coconut flour - .5 cup

Baking soda – 1 tsp.

Almond flour – 3 cups

Baking powder – 2 tsp.

Salt - .25 tsp.

Also Needed: Loaf pan – 9 x 5-inches

Directions:

Warm up the oven to 300ºF. Lightly spritz the pan with olive oil.

Combine all of the dry fixings and mix with the wet to prepare the dough.

Pour into the greased pan and bake for 1 hour.

Cool and slice.

182. Sesame Seed Bread

Servings: 6
Nutrition: 1 g Net Carbs ;7 g Proteins; 13 g Fat; 100 Calories
Ingredients:

Sesame seeds – 2 tbsp.

Psyllium husk powder – 5 tbsp.

Sea salt - .25 tsp.

Apple cider vinegar – 2 tsp.

Baking powder – 2 tsp.

Almond flour – 1.25 cups

Boiling water – 1 cup

Egg whites – 3

Directions:

Heat up the oven to reach 350ºF. Spritz a baking tin with some cooking oil spray. Put the water in a saucepan to boil.

Combine the psyllium powder, sesame seeds, sea salt, baking powder, and almond flour.

Stir in the boiled water, vinegar, and egg whites. Use a hand mixer (less than 1 min.to combine. Place the bread on the prepared pan.

Serve and enjoy any time after baking for 1 hour.

183. Spring Onion Bread

Servings: 6

Nutrition: 0.5 g Net Carbs; 2.2 g Proteins ;1.8 g Fat; 27 Calories

Ingredients:

Room temperature cream cheese – 3 tbsp.

Separated eggs – 3

Apple cider vinegar – 1 tbsp.

Minced spring onions – 3 tbsp.

Salt – to taste

Directions:

Warm up the oven to 300ºF.

Combine the whisked york with the spring onions and cream cheese.

In another container, whisk the salt, vinegar, and egg whites.

Prepare in batches, starting by adding the egg whites into the egg yolk mixture. Spoon the dough onto a parchment paper-lined pan. Be sure to leave room between each one. Bake for 20 minutes.

184. Stuffed Savory Bread

Nutrition: 2 g Net Carbs ; 6 g Proteins; 20 g Fat; 202 Calories

Ingredients:

Baking powder – 1.5 tsp.

Parsley seasoning – 2 tbsp.

Sage – 1 tsp

Rosemary – 1 tsp.

Medium eggs – 8

Cream cheese – 1 cup

Butter - .5 cup

Almond flour – 2.5 cups

Coconut flour - .25 cup

Directions:

Heat up the oven to 350F. Grease a loaf pan.

Cream/smash the butter and cream cheese. Fold in the seasonings (parsley, sage, and rosemary).

Whisk and break in the egg to form the batter until it's smooth.

Combine the almond and coconut flour with the baking powder, and add to the mixture until thick.

Scoop into the loaf pan and bake for 50 minutes. Serve and enjoy.

185. Garlic Breadsticks

Servings: 8 breadsticks

Nutrition: Calories: 259.2, Total Fat: 24.7 g, Saturated Fat: 7.5 g, Carbs: 6.3 g, Sugars: 1.1 g, Protein: 7 g

Ingredients for the garlic butter:

1/4 cup Butter, softened

1 tsp Garlic Powder

Ingredients:

2 cup Almond Flour

1/2 Tbsp Baking Powder

1 Tbsp Psyllium Husk Powder

1/4 tsp Salt

3 Tbsp Butter, melted

1 Egg

1/4 cup Boiling Water

Directions:

Preheat your oven to 400F / 200C.

Beat the garlic powder and butter and set aside to use it for brushing.

Combine the psyllium husk powder, baking powder, almond flour and salt. Add the butter along with the egg and mix until well combined.

Mix until dough forms using boiling water.

Divide into breadsticks.

Bake for 15 minutes. Brush the breadsticks with the garlic butter and bake for 5 more minutes.

Serve warm or allow to cool.

186. Savory Italian Crackers

Servings:20-30 crackers

Nutrition: Calories: 63.5, Total Fat: 5.8 g, Saturated Fat: 0.6 g, Carbs: 1.8 g, Sugars: 0.3 g, Protein: 2.1 g

Ingredients:

1 1/2 cup Almond Flour

1/4 tsp Garlic Powder

1/2 tsp Onion Powder

1/2 tsp Thyme

1/4 tsp Basil

1/4 tsp Oregano

3/4 tsp Salt

1 Egg

2 Tbsp Olive Oil

Directions:

Preheat your oven to 350F / 175C.

Combine until dough forms.

Form a log and slice into thin crackers. Arrange the crackers onto the prepared baking sheet and bake for about 10-15 minutes.

When done, allow to cool and serve.

187. Low-Carb Cream Cheese Rolls

Servings: 6 rolls

Nutrition:

Calorie 0.8 g Net Carbs ; 4.2 g Proteins; 8 g Fat; 91.3 Calories

Ingredients:

Large eggs – 3

Full-fat cream cheese - cubed & cold – 3 oz.

Cream of tartar - .125 tsp.

Salt - .125 tsp.

Directions:

Warm up the oven to 300ºF. Line a baking tin with parchment paper. Spritz the pan with cooking oil spray.

The yolks should separated from the eggs and place the whites in a non-greasy container. Whisk with the tartar until stiff.

In another container, whisk the cream cheese, salt, and yolks until smooth.

Fold in the whites of the eggs, mixing well using a spatula. Mound a scoop of whites over the yolk mixture and fold together as you rotate the dish. Continue the process until well combined. The process helps to eliminate the air bubbles.

Portion six large spoons of the mixture onto the prepared pan. Mash the tops with the spatulate to slightly flatten.

Bake until browned (30-40 min.).

Cool a few minutes in the pan. Then, carefully arrange them on a wire rack to cool.

Store in a zipper-type bag – open slightly – and store in the fridge for a couple of days for best results.

188. Homemade Sesame Breadsticks

 Nutrition:

Calories: 53.6, Total Fat: 5 g, Saturated Fat: 0.6 g, Carbs: 1.1 g, Sugars: 0.2 g, Protein: 1.6 g

Servings: 5 breadsticks

Ingredients:

1 Egg White

2 Tbsp Almond Flour

1 tsp Himalayan Pink Salt

1 Tbsp Extra Virgin Olive Oil

½ tsp Sesame Seeds

Directions:

Preheat your oven to 320F / 160C. Set aside after parchment paper is lined with the baking sheet.

Whisk the egg white and add the flour as well as half each the salt and olive oil.

Knead until you get smooth dough, divide into 5 pieces and roll into breadsticks.

Place on the prepared sheet, brush with the remaining olive oil, place the shee and sprinkle with the sesame seeds and the remaining salt.

Bake for about 20 minutes. Allow to cool slightly before serving.

189. Herb Bread

Nutrition:

Calories: 421, Total Fat: 37.4 g, Saturated Fat: 14.8 g, Carbs: 9.4 g, Sugars: 0.9 g, Protein: 15.1 g

Servings: 4

Ingredients:

2 Tbsp Coconut Flour

1 ½ cups Almond Flour

2 Tbsp Fresh Herbs of choice, chopped

2 Tbsp Ground Flax Seeds

1 ½ tsp Baking Soda

¼ tsp Salt

5 Eggs

1 Tbsp Apple Cider Vinegar

¼ cup Coconut Oil, melted

Directions:

Preheat your oven to 350F / 175C. Grease a loaf pan and set aside.

Add the coconut flour, almond flour, herbs, flax, baking soda, and salt to your food processor. Pulse to combine and then add the eggs, vinegar, and oil.

Transfer the batter to the prepared loaf pan and bake in the preheated oven for about half an hour.

Once baked and golden brown, remove from the oven, set aside to cool, slice and eat.

190. Almond Keto Bread

Nutrition:

Calories: 302, Total Fat: 28.6 g, Saturated Fat: 3 g, Carbs: 7.3g, Sugars: 1.2 g, Protein: 8.5 g

Servings: 10 slices

Ingredients:

3 cups Almond Flour

1 tsp Baking Soda

2 tsp Baking Powder

¼ tsp Salt

¼ cup Almond Milk

½ cup + 2 Tbsp Olive Oil

3 Eggs

Directions:

Preheat your oven to 300F / 149C. Grease a loaf pan (e.g. 9x5and set aside.

Combine all the ingredients and transfer the batter to the prepared loaf pan.

Bake in the preheated oven for an hour.

Once baked, remove from the oven, allow to cool, slice and eat.

191. Thanksgiving Bread

Nutrition:

Calories: 339, Total Fat: 26.9 g, Saturated Fat: 5.7 g, Carbs: 16.7 g, Sugars: 1.2 g, Protein: 12.2 g`

Servings: 4

Ingredients:

1 Tbsp Ghee

2 Celery Stalks, chopped

1 Onion, chopped

½ cup Walnuts

½ cup Coconut Flour

1½ cup Almond Flour

1 Tbsp Fresh Rosemary, chopped

10 Sage Leaves, finely chopped

1 tsp Baking Soda

1 pinch Freshly Grated Nutmeg

¼ tsp Salt

½ cup Chicken Broth

4 Eggs

2-3 Bacon Strips, cooked and crumbled

Directions:

Preheat your oven to 350F / 175C.

Add the ghee to a pan and melt on medium. Add the celery and onion and sauté for about 5 minutes.

Once tender, add the walnuts and cook for a few more minutes. Set aside.

In a bowl, mix together the coconut flour, almond flour, rosemary, sage, baking soda, nutmeg, and salt.

Mix in the sautéed celery and onion and add the chicken broth and eggs. Mix until well incorporated.

Stir in the bacon crumbles and transfer the batter to the prepared loaf pan. Bake n the preheated oven for about 30-35 minutes.

Once baked, leave to cool, slice and serve.

192. Hot Dog Rolls

Cooking time: 3 min

Servings: 3 buns

Nutrition facts: 274 calories per bun: Carbs 2.6g, fats 28.3g, and 7.8g proteins.

Ingredients:

6 oz almond flour

½ tbsp. baking powder

3 eggs

4 tbsp oil

salt

Steps:

Combine all the ingredients together: almond flour+ baking powder+eggs+oil+salt. Mix them well.

Microwave this mixture fo 1,5-2 min. Check it. If it is wet somewhere, microwave it for more 30 sec.

Cut from the bread the roll for your hot dogs.

Create the stuffing you like and enjoy.

193. Flax Tortillas

Servings: 5
Nutrition:
2.18 g Net Carbs ; 4.99 g Proteins; 11.78 g Fat; 184.4 Calories

Ingredients:
Golden flaxseed meal – 1 cup
Psyllium husk powder – 2 tbsp.
Olive oil – 2 tsp.
Xanthan gum - .25 tsp.
Curry powder - .5 tsp.
Filtered water - 1 cup (+2 tbsp.
Ingredients Per Tortilla:
Olive oil - for frying – 1 tsp
Coconut flour - for rolling - .5 tsp.

Directions:
Combine all of the dry fixings and add 2 teaspoons of oil and the water. Mix to form a dough. Let it rest uncovered for one hour on the countertop.

If cutting by hand, cut into 3 blocks. If you have a tortilla press, spit it into 5 chunks.

Press each portion with your hand and sprinkle with the coconut flour. Roll them out as thin as possible. Use a glass to cut out the tortillas. Re-roll any extra dough pieces.

Warm up the oil for frying and simmer over med-high heat for each of the tortillas.

194. Microwave Keto Bread

 Nutrition:

Calories: 357, Total Fat: 33.8 g, Saturated Fat: 11.6 g, Carbs: 6.4 g, Sugars: 1.2 g, Protein: 12.3 g

Servings: 4 slices

Ingredients:

⅓ cup Almond Flour

⅛ tsp Salt

½ tsp Baking Powder

2 ½ Tbsp Ghee, melted

1 Egg, whisked

Directions:

Grease a mug and set aside.

Combine all the ingredients to form a batter. Transfer to the greased mug and microwave for 90 seconds.

Leave to cool for several minutes.

Pop out of the mug, slice and eat.

195. Keto Rosemary Rolls

Cooking time: 20 min

Yield : 8 rolls

Nutrition facts: 89 calories per roll: Carbs 2.3g, fats 7.7g, and 3.3g proteins.

Ingredients:

2 tsp fresh rosemary

1 tbsp baking powder

4 oz cream cheese

3/4 cup mozzarella cheese, shredded

1 tsp dried chives

1 egg

1 cup almond flour

Steps:

Heat oven to 160°C.

Mix all dry ingredients: almond flour+baking powder+dried chives+fresh rosemary.

Microwave mozzarella+cream cheese for a minute.

Add there an egg and mix again.

Add to the egg with cheese mixed dry ingredients and make the dough.

Let it cool in a freezer for 15 min.

Oil your hands and form 8 small balls

Put them on a baking tray covered with the butter paper.

Bake for 20 min.

196. Keto Hot Dog Buns

Cooking time: 45 min

Servings: 10 rolls

Nutrition facts: 29 calories per roll: Carbs 1.5g, fats 2.1g, and 1.3g proteins.

Ingredients:

10 oz almond flour

1/3 cup psyllium husk powder

2 tsp baking powder

1 tsp sea salt

2 tsp cider vinegar

10 oz boiling water

3 egg whites

Steps:

Heat the oven to 175°C.

Mix all dry ingredients: almond flour+ psyllium husk powder+ baking powder+ sea salt.

Boil the water.

Add to dry ingredients: water+ vinegar+ egg whites and whisk. The dough should be soft.

Form 10 hot dog buns.

Put them on the baking tray covered with the butter paper.

Bake for 45 min.

Create the stuffing you like and enjoy.

197. Cloud Bread

Cooking time: 30 min

Servings: 8 clouds

Nutrition facts: 37 calories per cloud: Carbs 0.3g, fats 3g, and proteins 2.4g.

Ingredients:

1/4 tsp cream of tartar

3 eggs

3 tbsp cream cheese

Steps:

Heat the oven to 170 C.

Prepare the baking sheet.

Beat after separating the egg whotes from the york with tartar cream for 2-3 min using a hand mixer until stiff peaks.

Mix yolks and cream cheese separately.

Combine whites with yolks softly.

Form 8 mounds and place the dough onto the baking sheet, greased.

Bake for 30 min.

Intermediate

198. Coconut Bread Loaves

 Nutrition:

Calories: 297.5, Total Fat: 14.6 g, Saturated Fat: 2.6 g, Carbs: 25.5 g, Sugars: 0.3 g, Protein: 15.6 g

Servings: 4

Ingredients:

½ cup Ground Flax Seeds

½ tsp Baking Soda

1 tsp Baking Powder

1 tsp Salt

6 Eggs, room temperature

1 Tbsp Apple Cider Vinegar

½ cup Water

1 cup Coconut Flour, sifted

Directions:

Ensure that 350F / 175C is the target when preheating your oven. Grease a loaf pan and set aside.

Mix together the dry ingredients. Add in the water, eggs, and vinegar and mix well to incorporate.

Bake for 40 minutes.

When baked, leave to cool, slice and enjoy!

199. Soft Dinner Rolls

Cooking time: 20 min

Servings: 12 (2 rolls per serving

Nutrition facts: 157 calories per serving: Carbs 4.5g, fats 13.2g, and 6.6g proteins.

Ingredients:

10 oz almond flour

¼ cup baking powder

1 cup cream cheese

3 cups mozzarella, shredded

4 eggs

1 tbsp butter

Steps:

Heat the oven to 190°C

Microwave mozzarella+cream cheese for a minute.

Mix all dry ingredients: almond flour+baking powder+eggs

Add cheeses to dry ingredients, mix well and put aside for 15 min.

Form 12 rolls and let them cool in the freezer for 7-10 min.

Melt the butter in the iron skillet.

Put the rolls next to each other and bake for 20 min in the skillet.

Enjoy

Notes:

☐ So much quantity of baking powder will help the dough to rise well and not be flat.

200. Spicy Cloud Bread

Cooking time: 25-30 min

Servings: 6 clouds

Nutrition facts: 52 calories per cloud: Carbs 2.8g, fats 3.4g, and proteins 3.1g.

Ingredients:

3 eggs

4 tbsp xylitol

2 tbsp cream cheese

2 tsp cinnamon, ground

½ tsp baking powder

vanilla to taste

Steps:

Heat the oven to 175 C.

Prepare the baking sheet.

Beat the egg whites with baking powder for 2-3 min using a hand mixer until stiff peaks.

Mix yolks+cream cheese+vanilla+xylitol+cinnamon.

Combine whites with yolks softly.

Form 6 mounds and place the dough onto the baking sheet, greased. Make them flat.

Bake for 30 min until they are golden.

201. Avocado Cloud Bread

Cooking time: 30 min

Servings: 6 clouds

Nutrition facts: 76 calories per cloud: Carbs 1.8g, fats 6.2g, proteins 4g.

Ingredients:

1/4 tsp cream of tartar

4 eggs

½ avocado, mashed

Salt to taste

Seasoning for the top

Steps:

Heat the oven to 170 C.

Prepare the baking sheet.

Beat the egg whites with tartar cream for 2-3 min using a hand mixer until stiff peaks.

Combine yolks and avocado, mix well

Add whites to yolks softly.

Form 6 mounds and place the dough onto the baking sheet, greased. Make them flat.

Sprinkle them with seasoning.

Bake for 30 min until they are golden.

202. Keto Cheeseburger Muffin

Cooking time: 23 min

Servings: 9 muffins

Nutrition facts: 96 calories per muffin: Carbs 3.7g, fats 7g, and proteins 3.9g.

Ingredients:

8 tbsp almond flour

8 tbsp flaxseed meal

1 tsp baking powder

½ tspsalt

¼ tsp pepper

2 eggs

4 tbsp sour cream

Hamburger Filling:

1 lb ground beef

2 tbsp tomato paste

Salt, pepper,onion powder,garlic powder to taste

Toppings:

1.5 oz cheddar cheese

1 pickle, sliced

2 tbsp ketchup

2 tbsp mustard

Steps:

Heat the oven to 175 C.

Combine together: ground beef+seasoning+salt+pepper. Fry

Mix together the dry ingredients: almond flour+flaxseed meal+baking powder+salt+pepper.

Put there:sour cream+eggs

Place the dough into the baking silicone cups, greased. Leave some space at the top.

Put the ground beef on the top of the dough.

Bake for 20 min.

Take out of the oven and place the cheese on the ground beef. Bake for 3 min more.

Put the topping and enjoy.

203. Keto Flaxseed Cinnamon Bun Muffins

Cooking time: 15 min

Servings: 12 muffins

Nutrition facts: 209 calories per muffin: Carbs 7.1g, fats 16.8g, and proteins 5.8g.

Ingredients:

2 cups flaxseed meal

25 drops stevia

1 tbsp baking powder

2 tbsp cinnamon,ground

½ tbsp salt

5 eggs

½ cup water, room temperature

8 tbsp coconut oil, melted

2 tsp vanilla extract

Steps:

Heat the oven to 170 C.

Mix together dry ingredients: flaxseed meal+sweetener+baking powder+ cinnamon+salt.

Put together: eggs+ water+oil+vanilla extract. Blend for 30 sec. The mixture should be foamy.

Add dry mixture to the foamy and stir well.

Meanwhile prepare your silicone cups, grease them.

Put the dough into the cups. Approx. 4 tbsp per cup.

Bake for 15 min.

204. Keto-Bread Twists

Preparation time: 20 minutes

Cooking Time: 20 minutes

Servings: 6

Ingredients

¼ cup almond flour

2 Tbsp. coconut flour

½ tsp. salt

½ Tbsp. baking powder

½ cup cheese, shredded

2 Tbsp. butter

2 eggs

¼ cup green pesto

Directions:

Preheat the oven to 350F and prepare a baking tray.

Combine coconut flour, almond flour, baking powder, and salt in a bowl.

Mix butter, cheese, and egg in another bowl.

Combine the flour mixture with the butter mixture and form a dough.

Take 2 parchment sheets and place the dough in between them.

Form the dough into a rectangular shape with a rolling pin and remove the parchment paper from one side.

Drizzle the green pesto on the loaf and cut it into strips and twist them.

Put the baking tray in the oven and bake for 20 minutes.

Remove from oven and serve.

Nutrition:

Calories: 151

Fat: 12.9g

Carb: 3.5g

Protein: 5.8g

205. Keto Zucchini Toast

Preparation time: 15 minutes

Cooking Time: 20 minutes

Servings: 4

Ingredients

¼ cup almond flour

1 cup zucchini, shredded and boiled

¼ tsp. garlic powder

1 egg

1 Tbsp. flax meal

1 pinch black pepper

¼ tsp. oregano

1 pinch salt

¼ tsp. basil

Directions:

Preheat the oven to 450F and line a baking sheet with parchment paper.

Whisk the eggs with the rest of the ingredients in a bowl to form a batter.

Divide the batter into 4 equal parts and lay each on the baking sheet.

Transfer the sheet to the oven and bake for 20 minutes.

Remove, cool, and serve.

Nutrition:

Calories: 71

Fat: 5.1g

Carb: 3.2g

Protein: 3.6g

206. English Muffin

Preparation time: 10 minutes

Cooking Time: 5 minutes

Servings: 2

Ingredients

¼ cup almond flour

1 Tbsp. coconut flour

1/8 tsp. baking soda

1/8 tsp. salt

1 egg white

½ tsp. oil

2 Tbsp. warm water

Butter, jam, or scrambled egg for serving

Directions:

Add the flours, baking soda, and salt in a small ramekin and mix well with a fork.

Add the egg white, oil, and water, mix well.

Flatten the batter, so it is even on top.

Microwave the ramekin for 2 minutes.

Turn the ramekin upside down to slide out the muffin.

Slice it into 2 muffin halves and toast each slice.

Spread with butter or sugar-free jam or scrambled egg.

Serve.

Nutrition:

Calories: 114

Fat: 1g

Carb: 5g

Protein: 5g

207. Pumpkin Muffins

Preparation time: 10 minutes

Cooking Time: 15 minutes

Servings: 8

Ingredients

½ cup butternut squash or pumpkin puree

½ cup low carb sweetener

4 eggs

¼ tsp. baking soda

¼ tsp. salt

½ tsp. ground nutmeg

½ tsp. ground cinnamon

½ tsp. ground cloves

½ tsp. ground ginger

¼ cup plus 2 Tbsp. coconut flour

Directions:

Preheat the oven to 350F.

Prepare a muffin pan by lining the muffin wells with liners. Grease the liners.

Place the puree, sweetener, and eggs in a bowl and blend well. Mix with a mixer.

Add the salt, flour, baking soda, nutmeg, cinnamon, cloves, and ginger to the wet ingredients and mix well. Let the batter sit for a few minutes and then mix again.

Fill the muffin liners two-thirds full and bake for 15 minutes.

Cool and serve.

Nutrition:

Calories: 66

Fat: 3g

Carb: 6g

Protein: 4g

208. Chocolate Chip Muffins

Preparation time: 10 minutes

Cooking Time: 20 minutes

Servings: 8

Ingredients

½ cup coconut flour

¼ tsp. baking soda

¼ tsp. salt

4 eggs

1/3 cup unsalted butter, melted

½ cup low-carb sweetener

1 Tbsp. vanilla extract

2 Tbsp. coconut milk

1/3 cup sugar-free chocolate chips

Directions:

Preheat the oven to 350F.

Add the coconut flour, baking soda, and salt in a bowl and blend well.

Add the butter, eggs, sweetener, vanilla, and coconut milk to the dry ingredients and mix well. Gently stir in the chocolate chips.

Line muffin tins and fill ¾.

Bake for 20 minutes.

Cool and serve.

Nutrition:

Calories: 168

Fat: 13g

Carb: 6g

Protein: 5g

209. Blueberry Muffins

Preparation time: 10 minutes

Cooking Time: 20 minutes

Servings: 12

Ingredients

½ cup granulated sweetener Swerve

2 ½ cup almond flour

½ tsp. vanilla extract

¾ cup blueberries

1 ½ tsp. baking powder

1/3 cup almond milk, unsweetened

3 eggs

¼ tsp. salt

1/3 cup coconut oil, solid

Directions:

Preheat the oven to 350F. Line a cupcake pan with baking paper liners.

Mix the almond flour, baking powder, salt, and sweetener in a bowl.

Heat the coconut oil in a saucepan. Then put it slowly to the mixture of flour when melted.

Then mix the eggs, almond milk, and vanilla into the batter and mix.

Fold in the blueberries into the mixture.

Distribute the batter to the muffin cups.

Bake for 20 minutes.

Serve.

Nutritional Facts Per Serving

Calories: 125

Fat: 15g

Carb: 4g

Protein: 6g

210. Pepperoni Pizza

Preparation time: 5 minutes

Cooking Time: 10 minutes

Servings: 4

Ingredients

8 ounces mozzarella cheese, shredded

Garlic seasoning to taste

Italian herb seasoning to taste

2 ounces pepperoni, chopped

Directions:

Heat a non-stick skillet over medium heat.

When hot, sprinkle in the cheese in an even layer to cover the base of the skillet.

Sprinkle over the garlic and herb seasonings as soon as the cheese starts to bubble as well as the pepperoni.

When the edges of the pizza begin to brown, and it begins to loosen from the bottom of the skillet, slide the pizza out onto a serving plate.

Cool until firm.

Slice and serve.

Nutritional Facts Per Serving

Calories: 241

Fat: 17.6g

Carb: 2.2g

Protein: 17.9g

211. Pizza With A Chicken Crust

Preparation time: 10 minutes

Cooking Time: 20 minutes

Servings: 8

Ingredients

7 ounces chicken breast meat, ground

7 ounces mozzarella cheese, grated

1 tsp. garlic salt

1 tsp. dried basil

4 Tbsp. pizza topping sauce, no sugar added

4 ounces cheddar cheese, grated

12 slices pepperoni

Fresh basil leaves

Directions:

Pre-heat the oven to 450F.

Line a 12-inch pizza pan with parchment.

Mix the chicken, cheese, garlic salt, and dried basil together.

Spread into the pizza pan in an even layer and bake in the preheated oven for 10 to 12 minutes.

Remove from the oven and cool a little before adding the topping of sauce, cheddar cheese, and pepperoni.

Once the topping is on, replace it in the hot oven and cook for 5 to 7 minutes or until hot and bubbly.

Remove from the oven and top with torn basil leaves.

Cut and serve.

Nutrition:

Calories: 228

Fat: 14.6g

Carb: 3g

Protein: 20.2g

212. Keto Breakfast Pizza

Preparation time: 10 minutes

Cooking Time: 15 minutes

Servings: 2

Ingredients

½ tsp. salt

1 Tbsp. psyllium husk powder

2 cups cauliflower florets, riced

2 Tbsp. coconut flour

3 eggs

Directions:

Preheat the oven to 350F and line a baking tray with parchment paper.

In a bowl, add everything and mix well. Set aside for 5 minutes.

Then transfer into the baking tray. Flatten to give pizza dough shape.

Bake until golden brown, about 15 minutes.

Remove and top with toppings of your choice.

Serve.

Nutrition:

Calories: 454

Fat: 31g

Carb: 8g

Protein: 22g

213. Coconut & Psyllium Pizza Crust

Preparation time: 10 minutes

Cooking Time: 25 minutes

Servings: 4

Ingredients

¾ cup coconut flour

½ tsp. salt

½ tsp. baking soda

1 cup boiling water

1 tsp. powdered garlic

1 tsp. apple cider vinegar

3 eggs

3 Tbsp. psyllium husk powder

Directions:

Preheat the oven to 350F.

Combine the psyllium husk powder, coconut flour, salt, and powdered garlic in a bowl.

Add the baking soda, apple cider vinegar, and eggs into the mixing bowl and combine then pour in the boiling water and mix.

Spread out the dough on a parchment paper-lined baking sheet.

Bake for 15 to 20 minutes or until the edges start turning brown.

Top with cheese, sauce, and any other toppings of your choice and return into the oven until the cheese melts.

Serve warm.

Nutrition:

Calories: 189

Fat: 7g

Carb: 6g

Protein: 8g

214. Parmesan-Thyme Popovers

Preparation time: 10 minutes

Cooking Time: 15 minutes

Servings: 6

Ingredients

4 eggs

½ cup coconut milk

2 Tbsp. coconut flour

Pinch salt

1 Tbsp. parmesan cheese

1 Tbsp. chopped fresh thyme

Directions:

Preheat the oven to 425F.

Add all the ingredients to a bowl and whisk until fully blendedr.

Fill nonstick popover sleeves 2/3 with butter.

Bake for 15 minutes, or until they begin to brown on top.

Cool and serve.

Nutrition:

Calories: 64

Fat: 34g

Carb: 2g

Protein: 3g

215. Garlic-Cauliflower Breadsticks

Preparation time: 10 minutes

Cooking Time: 20 minutes

Servings: 16

Ingredients

2 cups grated cauliflower, riced

½ cup grated Parmesan cheese, divided

1 garlic clove, minced

¼ tsp. salt

2 tsp. chopped fresh herb

1 egg

2 Tbsp. coconut flour

½ cup marinara sauce

Directions:

Preheat the oven to 450F and line a baking sheet with parchment paper.

Steam the riced cauliflower for 5 minutes or until tender, but not soft.

Remove excess moisture from the steamed cauliflower with cheesecloth.

Add the cauliflower, ¼ cup cheese, garlic, salt, herbs, egg, and coconut flour in a bowl and mix well.

On parchment paper, shape the mixture into a rectangle about ½ inch thick.

Bake the breadsticks for 15 minutes, or until the edges begin to brown.

Brush the top with marinara sauce and sprinkle the remaining ¼-cup cheese.

Place back in the oven and bake until the cheese starts to brown.

Cool, slice, and serve.

Nutrition:

Calories: 63

Fat: 4g

Carb: 1g

Protein: 5g

216. Spring Onion Buns

Servings: 6

Calories: 81
Fat: 6.7 g
Protein: 4.2 g
Carbs: 1.1 g
Ingredients
3 eggs, separated
3 1/2 oz. cream cheese
1 tsp. stevia
1/2 tsp. baking powder
Salt, to taste
For Filling:
1 egg, hard boiled, chopped
2 sprigs spring onions, chopped
Direction
Combine egg yolks with stevia, cream cheese, baking powder and salt.
Whisk egg whites until foamy.
Using a spatula mix the egg whites into the yolk mixture.
Pour the dough into greased muffin cups filling ½ of the cup.
Combine spring onions with chopped egg and add this filling to muffin cups.
Pour more dough into the cups.
Bake at 300°F for 30 minutes. Serve and enjoy!

217. Sesame Buns

Servings: 12

Calories: 133

Fat: 6.5 g

Protein: 6.9 g

Carbs: 4 g

Ingredients

6 egg whites

1 cup coconut flour

1 tsp. baking powder

1 cup sesame seeds, separated (1/2 cup for the dough, 1/2 cup for coating

1/2 cup pumpkin seeds

1/2 cup psyllium powder

1 cup hot water

Salt, to taste

Direction

Combine all dry ingredients except ½ cup of sesame seeds.

Whisk the egg whites until foamy.

Add foamy whites to dry ingredients, give a good stir.

Add 1 cup boiling water slowly, constantly stirring.

Put the remaining ½ cup sesame seeds in a separate bowl.

With your hands, shape the buns round and coat in sesame seeds.

Line a baking sheet with parchment paper and place the buns on it.

Bake at 350 degrees F for 50 minutes. Serve and enjoy!

218. Protein Buns

Servings: 8

Calories: 29

Fat: 0.3 g

Protein: 6.4 g

Carbs: 0.1 g

Ingredients

2 eggs

1/2 cup water

1 1/2 to 2 oz. soya protein powder

1 dash Stevia or to taste

Cinnamon or vanilla extract, to taste

Direction

Whisk the eggs and then add other ingredients. Then whisk well.

Divide between 8 greased silicone cups and bake at 430 degrees F for 20 minutes.

Lower the temperature to 340 degrees F and bake for 10 to 15 minutes more. Serve and enjoy!

219. Sandwich Buns

Servings: 7

Calories: 99

Fat: 6 g

Protein: 5.3 g

Carbs: 10 g

Ingredients

4 eggs

2 1/2 oz. almond flour

1 tbsp. coconut flour

1 oz. psyllium

1 1/2 cups eggplants, finely grated, juices drained

3 tbsp. sesame seeds

1 1/2 tsp. baking powder

Salt, to taste

Direction

Whisk eggs until foamy, and then add grated eggplant.

In a separate bowl mix all dry ingredients.

Add them to the egg mixture. Mix well.

Line a baking sheet with parchment paper and shape the buns with your hands.

Bake at 374°F for 20–25 minutes. Serve and enjoy!

220. Flax Seed Buns

Servings: 6

Calories: 85

Fat: 5 g

Protein: 5.9 g

Carbs: 7 g

Ingredients

1 egg

2 egg whites

1 3/4 oz. flax seed

1 3/4 oz. (1/2 cupoat bran, ground

1 3/4 oz. buttermilk

1 tsp. baking powder

Salt, to taste

Direction

Combine dry ingredients.

Add 1 egg and 2 egg whites and then mix well.

Now add the buttermilk and whisk.

Spoon the dough into muffin cups and bake at 356 degrees F for 20 minutes. Serve and enjoy!

221. Swedish Tea Buns

Servings: 6 tea buns

Calories: 313

Fat: 22.7 g

Protein: 10.5 g

Carbs: 8 g

Fiber: 1.1 g

Ingredients

100 g butter

6 eggs

3/4 cup almond flour

1/2 cup coconut flour

1 tsp. baking powder

1/2 tsp. salt

Direction

Preheat the oven to 375F.

Melt butter and line a baking sheet with parchment paper.

Beat eggs with a hand mixer and add melted, and cooled butter and mix well.

In another bowl, mix dry ingredients, then blend thoroughly into the batter.

Set aside for 10 minutes.

Space 6 mounds well apart on the baking sheet.

With a wet spoon, flatten the mounds into round buns, about half an inch.

Bake in the middle of the oven for 20 minutes.

Cool and serve. Enjoy!

222. Gluten-Free Low Carb Keto Buns

Servings: 14

Calories: 299

Fat: 24.9 g

Protein: 9.3 g

Carbs: 1.4 g

Fiber: 0.4 g

Ingredients

1 tbsp. butter

1 egg

1 tbsp. coconut milk

1 tbsp. almond meal

1 tbsp. coconut flour

1/8 tsp. baking soda

Sesame seeds, for topping

Direction

In a bowl, mix the butter, egg, coconut milk, almond meal, coconut flour and the baking soda.

Pour the batter in to a greased cake pan.

Sprinkle sesame seeds from the top and bake in preheated oven at 350 degrees Fahrenheit for about a minute.

Cut when the bread cools down and serve. Enjoy!

223. Almond Buns

Servings: 3

Total Time: 5 Minutes

Calories: 152

Fat: 24 g

Protein: 11 g

Carbs: 1.5 g

Fiber: 2 g

Ingredients

3/4 cup almond flour

2 eggs

5 tbsp. butter

1 1/2 tbsp. splenda

1 1/2 tsp. baking powder

Direction

Mix together the sweetener, splenda, baking powder and the almond flour.

Now mix in the eggs.

Next, melt the butter and put in the mixture.

Pour the mixture equally in to greased muffin cups.

Preheat your oven at 350 degrees Fahrenheit.

Put the muffin tray in the preheated oven to bake for 15 to 17 minutes or until done.

Serve when cool. Enjoy!

224. Keto Basil Buns

Servings: 8

Calories: 186

Fat: 15 g

Protein: 9.6 g

Carbs: 1.4 g

Ingredients

4 eggs

3/4 cup almond flour

6 tbsp. butter

6 tbsp. butter

6 garlic cloves, crushed

5 1/2 oz. parmesan cheese, grated

3/4 cup water

1 cup fresh basil, chopped

Salt, to taste

Direction

Heat water until boiling and add butter and salt.

Add flour and mix until smooth. Then remove from the heat.

Crack eggs into the dough one at a time, mixing after each egg.

Add basil, garlic and, last, the Parmesan. Mix until smooth.

Line a baking sheet with parchment paper and place the dough on it one spoonful at a time to form buns.

Bake at 392°F for 20 minutes. Serve and enjoy!

225. Keto Basil Buns

Servings: 8

Calories: 91
Fat: 4.2 g
Protein: 3.3 g
Carbs: 12.1 g
Ingredients
2 egg whites
1 cup sunflower seeds, ground
1/4 cup flax seeds, ground
5 tbsp. psyllium husks
1 cup water, hot
2 tsp. baking powder
Salt, to taste
Direction
Combine all dry ingredients.
Add egg whites and using a blender, whisk until smooth.
Add boiling water and keep whisking.
Line a baking sheet with parchment paper and drop the dough on it one spoonful at a time to form buns.
Bake at 356°F for 50 minutes. Serve and enjoy!

226. Coconut Cookies

Servings: 12

Calories: 144

Fat: 10.4 g

Protein: 1.4 g

Carbs: 30 g

Ingredients

2 egg whites

1 1/2 cups coconut flakes

1/2 stick (2 oz.butter, melted, cooled

2 tbsp. coconut flour

1 cup erythritol

Direction

Combine flour, coconut flakes and erythritol.

Add egg whites and melted butter. Give a good stir.

Line a baking sheet with parchment paper and put the cookie batter on it by the spoonsful.

Bake at 392 degrees F for 7 minutes. Serve and enjoy!

227. Coconut Balls

Servings: 12

Calories: 144

Fat: 55 g

Protein: 20.3 g

Carbs: 6 g

Ingredients

3 egg whites

1 tbsp. coconut flakes

2 1/2 oz. coconut flakes

Sweetener of your choice, to taste

Direction

Whisk egg whites until foamy.

Combine flour with coconut flakes and add to egg foam. Mix with a spoon, not a blender.

Shape into balls and place on a baking sheet lined with parchment paper.

Bake at 392 degrees F for 15 minutes. Serve and enjoy!

228. Apple Carrot Cookies

Servings: 10

Calories: 29

Fat: 0.6 g

Protein: 0.9 g

Carbs: 5.4 g

Ingredients

1 apple, peeled, grated

1 carrot, grated

1 egg white

4 tbsp. oatmeal

1/2 tsp. cinnamon

Handful raisins

1 tsp. stevia

Direction

Combine all ingredients and give a good stir.

Line a baking sheet with parchment paper and spoon the cookies onto it.

Bake at 392 degrees F for 20 to 30 minutes. Serve and enjoy!

229. Cream Cheese Cookies

Servings: 10

Calories: 106
Fat: 9 g
Protein: 3 g
Carbs: 3 g
Ingredients
1 egg white
1/4 cup butter, soft
3 cups almond flour
2 oz. cream cheese
2 tsp. vanilla extract
3/4 cup erythritol
Direction
Beat together the butter, cream cheese and erythritol.
Add vanilla and egg white.
Gradually sift flour, ½ cup at a time into the mixture.
Line a baking sheet with parchment paper and spoon the cookies onto it.
Bake at 350 degrees F for 15 minutes. Serve and enjoy!

230. Crispy Keto Cookies

Servings: 12

Calories: 104

Fat: 2.1 g

Protein: 12.3 g

Carbs: 11 g

Ingredients

2 eggs

1 tbsp. soy flour

3 tbsp. oat bran

1 to 2 tsp. coconut chips

1/2 cup milk

Dash of baking soda

Vanilla extract, to taste

Sweetener of your choice, to taste

Direction

Combine all ingredients and allow to stand for 15 minutes. The dough will be watery but this is OK.

Pour the dough into silicone molds, about 1 tbsp. into each.

Bake at 390 degrees for 15 to 20 minutes. Serve and enjoy!

231. Ginger Cookies

Servings: 10

Calories: 21

Fat: 1.1 g

Protein: 1.6 g

Carbs: 2.4 g

Ingredients

3 tbsp. oat bran

2 egg whites

1 tbsp. dried ginger

1 tsp. plain cow's milk yogurt

1 tsp. baking powder

Sweetener of your choice, to taste

Direction

Combine all ingredients. Add more bran if the dough is too runny. Then mix well.

Line a baking sheet with parchment paper and spoon the cookies onto it.

Bake at 356 degrees F for 15 minutes. Serve and enjoy!

232. Oatmeal Cookies

Servings: 15

Calories: 51

Fat: 0.9 g

Protein: 2.5 g

Carbs: 8.6 g

Ingredients

3 eggs

2 cups oat flakes, ground

1/3 tsp. vanilla extract

Dash of cinnamon

2 tsp. erythritol

Direction

Whisk eggs and add vanilla extract.

In a separate bowl, combine oatmeal, erythritol and cinnamon.

Add the egg mixture and combine.

Line a baking sheet with parchment paper and put the cookie batter on it by spoonsful.

Bake at 392°F for 15–20 minutes. Serve and enjoy!

233. Oatmeal Banana Cookies

Servings: 10

Calories: 120
Fat: 1.2 g
Protein: 5.2 g
Carbs: 6 g
Ingredients
8 oz. cottage cheese, fat free
1 cup oatmeal
1 apple, peeled, cored, grated
1 banana
1 tbsp. lemon juice
1 tsp. honey
Direction
Mix the cottage cheese with the honey and oatmeal.
Combine grated apple with lemon juice.
Mash the banana with a fork.
Mix all ingredients together.
Line a baking sheet with parchment paper and spoon the cookies onto it.
Bake at 392 degrees F for 30 minutes. Serve and enjoy!

234. Oat Sticks

Servings: 10

Calories: 137
Fat: 10.2 g
Protein: 4 g
Carbs: 7.5 g
Ingredients
1 cup oat flakes, finely ground
2 1/2 oz. butter, cubed
2 oz. cheese of your choice, grated
1 cup milk
1/2 cup almond flour
Salt, to taste
Direction
Combine oat flakes, flour and salt.
Add butter, milk and grated cheese and mix thoroughly.
Knead the dough. It will be thick.
Roll out the dough about ¼ inch thick with a rolling pin, and cut into sticks.
Line a baking sheet with parchment paper and place the sticks on it.
Bake at 380° F for 12 minutes. Serve and enjoy!

235. Simple Keto Cookies

Servings: 10

Calories: 137

Fat: 10.2 g

Protein: 4 g

Carbs: 7.5 g

Ingredients

2 cups flakes of your choice (oat or buckwheat or a mix of the two

1 eggs

2 cups water

Sweetener of your choice, to taste

Direction

Dissolve the sweetener in water and add the flakes.

Let soak for 10 minutes. Add more water if needed.

Add an egg and mix well.

Line a baking sheet with parchment paper and shaping by hand, place the cookies on the paper.

Bake at 380 degrees F for 20 minutes. Serve and enjoy!

236. Pumpkin Almond Cookies

Servings: 12

Calories: 315

Fat: 20 g

Protein: 8.3 g

Carbs: 26 g

Ingredients

1 egg white

1 cup pumpkin puree

1 cup almond flour

1 cup almonds, ground

2 tbsp. maple syrup

1/4 cup coconut flakes

1/4 cup lemon zest, grated

Direction

Combine flour, almonds, coconut flakes and lemon zest.

In a separate bowl whisk egg white until foamy.

Gradually add maple syrup.

Mix all ingredients together with pumpkin purée.

Line a baking sheet with parchment paper and add the cookies by the spoonful.

Bake at 302°F for 30 minutes. Serve and enjoy!

Buns

Chapter 5. Gluten Free Loaves

237. Gingerbread Spiced Bundt Cake

PREPARATION TIME: 15 MINUTES, PLUS 1 HOUR TO SET

COOKING TIME: 60 TO 70 MINUTES

SERVINGS: 12

For the cake

1½ cups molasses

1 cup hot (not boilingwater

2 cups garbanzo bean flour

1 cup almond meal

1 cup brown rice flour

3 tablespoons psyllium husk

1 tablespoon ground ginger

2 teaspoons baking soda

1 teaspoon ground cinnamon

½ teaspoon ground nutmeg

½ teaspoon ground cloves

½ teaspoon salt

1 cup vegan butter, at room temperature

1 cup packed light brown sugar or coconut sugar

3 large eggs

1 teaspoon vanilla extract

For the glaze

1 cup confectioners' sugar

1 to 2 tablespoons unsweetened dairy-free milk

¼ teaspoon vanilla extract

1.For the cake, preheat the oven to 350°F. Lightly coat a 9-inch Bundt pan with nonstick cooking spray and dust with garbanzo bean flour. In a large liquid measuring cup, combine the molasses and water.

2.In a medium bowl, combine the garbanzo bean flour, almond meal, rice flour, psyllium husk, ginger, baking soda, cinnamon, nutmeg, cloves, and salt.

3.In a large bowl, using an electric mixer on medium speed, cream the butter and sugar together. On low speed, beat in the eggs and vanilla until combined. Add half the flour mixture and stir with a spatula until incorporated. Add the molasses-water mixture and remaining flour mixture and stir until smooth and creamy. Pour the batter into the prepared pan.

4.Bake until a toothpick inserted in the center comes out clean, about 60 to 70 minutes. Let cool for 30 minutes on a wire rack, then turn out of the pan onto the rack to cool completely.

5.For the glaze, 1 hour before serving, in a small bowl, whisk together the sugar, milk, and vanilla until smooth. Drizzle over the cake. Let stand for 1 hour until set.

PREP TIP: Allowing the cake to cool in the pan for 30 minutes helps the cake settle and hold its shape. To remove it from the pan, run a knife around the edge to loosen before turning the cake out onto the rack.

STORAGE: Store at room temperature in an airtight container for up to 3 days.

SUBSTITUTIONS: You can swap 3½ cups gluten-free flour blend for the flours, but it will yield a slightly drier cake.

238. Angel Food Cake with Coconut Whipped Cream and Strawberries

PREPARATION TIME: 30 MINUTES

COOKING TIME: 45 MINUTES

SERVINGS: 12

For the cake

1½ cups granulated sugar, divided

¾ cup sweet white rice flour

½ cup potato starch

¼ cup tapioca flour

2 teaspoons xanthan gum

12 large egg whites, at room temperature

1½ teaspoons vanilla extract

¼ teaspoon almond extract

½ teaspoon salt

1 teaspoon cream of tartar

For the coconut whipped cream and strawberries

1 (13.5-ouncecan coconut cream or full-fat coconut milk, chilled for 24 hours

½ cup confectioners' sugar

½ teaspoon vanilla extract

4 cups sliced strawberries

For the cake, preheat the oven to 325°F. Do not grease the angel food cake pan.

Sift ¾ cup of the sugar, the rice flour, potato starch, tapioca flour, and xanthan gum into a medium bowl.

In a large bowl, using an electric mixer on medium-high speed, beat the egg whites, vanilla, almond extract, and salt together until foamy. Add the cream of tartar and beat until soft peaks form. Continue beating while gradually add the remaining sugar, ¼ cup at a time, until incorporated. Continue to beat until stiff, glossy peaks form.

Sift one-third of the flour mixture over the egg white mixture. Carefully fold it in with a spatula until incorporated. Repeat this process twice with the remaining flour mixture. Pour the batter into the pan. Run a knife through the center of the batter to release any air bubbles. Smooth the top with a spatula for even baking.

Bake until the top is lightly golden and cracked and a toothpick inserted in the center comes out with just a few crumbs, 35 to 45 minutes. Turn the pan upside down on a wire rack, the neck of a tall wine bottle, or the feet of the pan (if it has them). Let cool completely for 2 hours. Run a knife carefully around the inside edge of the pan to loosen the cake, then turn it out onto a wire rack.

For the coconut whipped cream, turn the can of coconut cream upside down to open. Drain and discard the water. Scoop the cream into a large bowl. Using an electric mixer on high speed, beat until it has the consistency of whipped cream, about 5 minutes. Add the sugar and vanilla and beat for 1 minute, until blended.

Slice and serve the angel food cake with a dollop of whipped cream topped with the strawberries.

PREP TIPS:

Make sure not to grease the pan, because the fat will deflate the egg whites.

If you use a stand mixer, use the whisk attachment to beat the eggs.

When folding the flour into the eggs, be sure not to stir too vigorously, or you will deflate the egg whites.

239. Lemon-Raspberry Quick Bread

PREPARATION TIME: 15 MINUTES, PLUS OVERNIGHT TO SET
COOKING TIME: 1 HOUR
SERVINGS: 12

¾ cup sweet white rice flour

½ cup sorghum flour

¼ cup potato starch

1 tablespoon baking powder

1½ teaspoons xanthan gum

Grated zest of 2 large lemons (2 teaspoons)

½ teaspoon baking soda

¼ teaspoon salt

1 cup granulated sugar

2 large eggs

½ cup vegan butter, melted

½ cup vanilla dairy-free yogurt

2 tablespoons freshly squeezed lemon juice

½ teaspoon lemon extract (optional)

1½ cups raspberries

Preheat the oven to 350°F. Line a 9-inch loaf pan with parchment paper so there is an overhang on two sides.

In a medium bowl, combine the rice flour, sorghum flour, potato starch, baking powder, xanthan gum, lemon zest, baking soda, and salt.

In a large bowl, whisk together the sugar, eggs, butter, yogurt, lemon juice, and lemon extract (if using). Stir in the flour mixture just until moistened. Carefully fold in the raspberries. Spoon the batter into the prepared pan.

Bake until a toothpick inserted in the center comes out clean, about 1 hour, covering with aluminum foil after 45 minutes of baking. Let cool on a wire rack for 20 minutes, then use the parchment paper to lift it from the baking pan and transfer to the rack to cool completely. Wrap and store overnight for best slicing.

PREP TIP: Carefully fold in the raspberries, or they will break, turning the bread pink.

STORAGE: Store the loaf whole, tightly wrapped in a piece of aluminum foil lined with wax paper. Once sliced, store at room temperature in an airtight container for up to 3 days. Or freeze the foil-wrapped loaf or slices in a zip-top plastic bag for up to 3 months.

240. Pumpkin Quick Bread

PREPARATION TIME: 15 MINUTES, PLUS OVERNIGHT TO SET

COOKING TIME: 55 MINUTES

SERVINGS: 12

1⅓ cups Basic Gluten-Free Flour Blend or store-bought equivalent

2 teaspoons baking soda

1 teaspoon ground nutmeg

1 teaspoon ground cinnamon

1 teaspoon salt

1 (15-ouncecan pumpkin purée (not pumpkin pie filling)

1 cup packed light brown sugar or coconut sugar

4 large eggs

Preheat the oven to 350°F. Line a 9-inch loaf pan with parchment paper so there is an overhang on two sides.

In a medium bowl, combine the flour blend, baking soda, nutmeg, cinnamon, and salt.

In a large bowl, using an electric mixer on medium speed, beat the pumpkin purée and sugar together until blended. Beat in the eggs until well combined. On low speed, add the flour mixture in three additions, beating just until combined. Spoon into the prepared pan.

Bake until a toothpick inserted in the center comes out clean, 50 to 55 minutes. Let cool on a wire rack for 20 minutes, then remove the bread by lifting the parchment paper. Transfer to the rack and let cool completely. Wrap and store overnight for best slicing.

PREP TIP: Check the bread for burning after 40 minutes, and, if needed, cover lightly with foil to finish baking.

STORAGE: Store the loaf whole, tightly wrapped in a piece of aluminum foil lined with wax paper. Once sliced, store at room temperature in an airtight container for up to 3 days. Or freeze the foil-wrapped loaf or slices in a zip-top plastic bag for up to 3 months.

241. Banana-Nut Bread

PREPARATION TIME: 15 MINUTES, PLUS OVERNIGHT TO SET
COOKING TIME: 55 MINUTES
SERVINGS: 12

3 ripe bananas

2 cups Basic Gluten-Free Flour Blend or store-bought equivalent

1 tablespoon baking powder

1 teaspoon ground cinnamon

½ teaspoon salt

⅛ teaspoon ground ginger

2 large eggs

⅔ cup maple syrup

½ cup plain dairy-free yogurt

1 tablespoon vanilla extract

¾ cup chopped walnuts, divided

Preheat the oven to 350°F. Line a 9-inch loaf pan with parchment paper so there is an overhang on two sides.

In a small bowl with a fork, mash the bananas until creamy and blended.

In a medium bowl, combine the flour blend, baking powder, cinnamon, salt, and ginger.

In a large bowl, using an electric mixer on medium speed, beat the eggs, maple syrup, yogurt, and vanilla together until well blended. Beat in the mashed bananas until combined. On low speed, beat in the flour mixture just until combined. Fold in ½ cup of walnuts. Spoon the batter into the prepared pan. Sprinkle the remaining ¼ cup of walnuts over the top.

Bake until a toothpick inserted in the center comes out clean, 50 to 55 minutes. Let cool on a wire rack for 20 minutes, then remove the bread by lifting the parchment paper. Transfer to the rack and let cool completely.

STORAGE: Store the loaf whole, tightly wrapped in a piece of aluminum foil lined with wax paper. Once sliced, store at room temperature in an airtight container for up to 3 days. Or freeze the foil-wrapped loaf or slices in a zip-top plastic bag up to 3 months.

242. Cherry, Orange, and Pistachio Quick Bread with Orange Glaze

PREPARATION TIME: 15 MINUTES, PLUS OVERNIGHT TO SET

COOKING TIME: 55 MINUTES

SERVINGS: 12

For the cake

2 cups Basic Gluten-Free Flour Blend or store-bought equivalent

1 tablespoon baking powder

Grated zest of 2 oranges (2 teaspoons)

½ teaspoon salt

2 large eggs

½ cup maple syrup

¾ cup freshly squeezed orange juice

¼ cup avocado oil

1 cup coarsely chopped pitted fresh cherries

¾ cup chopped pistachios

For the glaze

1 cup confectioners' sugar

1 to 2 tablespoons freshly squeezed orange juice

Grated zest of 1 orange (1 teaspoon)

For the cake, preheat the oven to 350°F. Line a 9-inch loaf pan with parchment paper so there is an overhang on two sides.

In a medium bowl, combine the flour blend, baking powder, orange zest, and salt.

In a large bowl, whisk the eggs, maple syrup, orange juice, and oil. Stir in the flour mixture just until combined. Carefully fold in the cherries and pistachios. Spoon into the prepared pan.

Bake until a toothpick inserted in the center comes out clean, 50 to 55 minutes. Let cool on a wire rack for 20 minutes, then remove the bread by lifting the parchment paper. Transfer to the rack to cool completely. Wrap and store overnight for best slicing.

For the glaze, 1 hour before serving, in a small bowl, whisk together the sugar, orange juice, and zest until smooth. Drizzle over the bread. Let stand for 1 hour until set.

STORAGE: Store the loaf whole, tightly wrapped in a piece of aluminum foil lined with wax paper. Once sliced, store at room temperature in an airtight container for up to 3 days. Or freeze the foil-wrapped loaf or slices in a zip-top plastic bag for up to 3 months.

SUBSTITUTIONS: Use fresh cranberries instead of the cherries.

243. Lemon–Poppy Seed Bread

PREPARATION TIME: 15 MINUTES, PLUS OVERNIGHT TO SET
COOKING TIME: 55 MINUTES
SERVINGS: 12

1¾ cups Basic Gluten-Free Flour Blend or store-bought equivalent

¼ cup potato starch

1 tablespoon baking powder

Grated zest of 2 large lemons (2 teaspoons)

1½ teaspoons xanthan gum

½ teaspoon salt

3 large eggs

½ cup vegan butter, at room temperature

1 cup honey

⅓ cup plain dairy-free yogurt

¼ cup freshly squeezed lemon juice

½ teaspoon vanilla extract

1 teaspoon lemon extract

1 tablespoon poppy seeds

Preheat the oven to 350°F. Lightly coat a 9-inch loaf pan with nonstick cooking spray.

In a medium bowl, combine the flour blend, potato starch, baking powder, lemon zest, xanthan gum, and salt.

In a large bowl, whisk together the eggs, butter, honey, yogurt, lemon juice, vanilla, and lemon extract. Stir in the flour mixture just until combined. Fold in the poppy seeds just until blended. Spoon the batter into the prepared pan.

Bake until a toothpick inserted in the center comes out clean, 50 to 55 minutes. Let cool on a wire rack for 20 minutes, then remove the bread from the pan and place it on the rack to cool completely. Wrap and store overnight for best slicing.

PREP TIP: Be careful not to overmix, or the poppy seeds will brown the batter.

STORAGE: Store the loaf whole, tightly wrapped in a piece of aluminum foil lined with wax paper. Once sliced, store at room temperature in an airtight container for up to 3 days. Or freeze the foil-wrapped loaf or slices in a zip-top plastic bag up to 3 months.

244. Skillet Corn Bread

PREPARATION TIME: 15 MINUTES

COOKING TIME: 30 MINUTES

SERVINGS: 8

2 cups white or yellow cornmeal

½ cup Basic Gluten-Free Flour Blend or store-bought equivalent

½ cup tapioca flour

3 tablespoons psyllium husk

1 tablespoon baking powder

1½ teaspoons xanthan gum

½ teaspoon salt

¼ teaspoon baking soda

2 large eggs

½ cup vegan butter, at room temperature

½ cup honey

2 tablespoons molasses

1½ to 2 cups unsweetened dairy-free milk

Preheat the oven to 375°F. Lightly coat a 9-inch cast iron skillet with nonstick cooking spray.

In a medium bowl, combine the cornmeal, flour blend, tapioca flour, psyllium husk, baking powder, xanthan gum, salt, and baking soda.

In large bowl, using an electric mixer on medium speed, beat the eggs, butter, honey, molasses, and 1½ cups of milk together until well mixed. Stir in the flour mixture just until combined. The batter should be smooth with a cake batter consistency. Add additional milk, 1 tablespoon at a time, if necessary. Pour the batter into the prepared skillet.

Bake until the top is golden brown and a toothpick inserted in the center comes out with just a few crumbs, about 30 minutes. Let cool for 5 minutes before cutting into wedges and serving directly from the pan.

STORAGE: Store at room temperature in an airtight container for up to 3 days.

SUBSTITUTIONS: This cornbread can be turned into muffins. Spoon the batter into a 12-cup muffin pan lined with paper cups that have been lightly coated with nonstick cooking spray. Bake for 20 to 28 minutes.

245. SWEET AND SAVORY PIES AND FRUIT DESSERTS

Basic Gluten-Free Pie Dough

Sweet Tart Dough

Double-Crusted Berry Pie

Marbled Chocolate and Peanut Butter Pie

Key Lime Pie

Pumpkin Pie

Blackberry Galette

Double Chocolate Tart with Raspberries and Coconut Whipped Cream

Summer Vegetable Tart

Bacon, Mushroom, and Thyme Quiche

Spinach and Sun-Dried Tomato Potato-Crusted Quiche

Chicken-Mushroom Pot Pie

Warm Peach Cobbler

Apple-Cranberry Crumble

Coconut-Raisin Baked Rice Pudding

T hese simple pies, tarts, and quiches are luscious, elegant, and a beautiful addition to any table. I hope you celebrate summer with a blackberry galette and key lime pie, fill the holiday season with pumpkin pie and fruit crumble, and end a long weekend with the luxury of an easy savory quiche. Pies take time and more effort than other baked goods, but they are worth the work with every flaky, satisfying bite. In addition, I've included recipes for cobblers, crisps, and rice pudding—some of the most comforting of desserts.

246. Basic Gluten-Free Pie Dough

PREPARATION TIME: 10 MINUTES, PLUS 30 MINUTES TO CHILL
SERVINGS: 2 (9-INCHPIE CRUSTS OR 1 (9-INCHDOUBLE CRUST

1 large egg

½ teaspoon apple cider vinegar

¼ cup ice water

2 cups Gluten-Free Cake and Pastry Flour Blend or store-bought equivalent

1 teaspoon granulated sugar

1 teaspoon xanthan gum

¾ teaspoon salt

¾ cup vegan butter, cut into 1-tablespoon slices and frozen for 10 minutes

In a small bowl, whisk the egg, vinegar, and water together.

In a large bowl, sift the flour blend, sugar, xanthan gum, and salt together. Using a pastry blender or two knives, cut in the butter until crumbly with pea-size chunks. With a fork, stir in the egg mixture until the dough is moist and can be formed into a ball.

Divide the dough into two disks, wrap each in plastic wrap, and refrigerate for 30 minutes or until ready to use. Use as directed in the individual recipe.

PREP TIP: Freezing the butter for 10 minutes before using will result in a flakier piecrust.

STORAGE: Store the wrapped disks in the refrigerator for up to 3 days or in a zip-top plastic bag in the freezer up to 1 month. Thaw in the refrigerator overnight before using.

247. Sweet Tart Dough

PREPARATION TIME: 10 MINUTES, PLUS 30 MINUTES TO CHILL
SERVINGS: 3 (9-INCHTART SHELLS

3 cups Gluten-Free Cake and Pastry Flour Blend or store-bought equivalent

¼ cup tapioca flour

⅓ cup maple syrup

1½ teaspoons xanthan gum

½ teaspoon apple cider vinegar

1½ cups vegan butter, cubed and frozen for 10 minutes

¼ cup ice water

In a food processor, pulse the flour blend, tapioca flour, maple syrup, xanthan gum, vinegar, and butter together until it forms coarse crumbs. Add the ice water and pulse again until fine crumbs form. Be careful not to overmix.

Transfer the dough to a floured work surface and knead until it forms a ball. Divide into three portions. Form each portion into a disk, wrap in plastic, and refrigerate for 30 minutes before using. Use as directed in the individual recipe.

PREP TIP: Take care not to overmix. You want the dough to resemble small crumbs before being formed into disks.

STORAGE: Store the wrapped disks in the refrigerator for up to 3 days or in a zip-top plastic bag in the freezer up to 1 month. Thaw in the refrigerator overnight before using.

248. Double-Crusted Berry Pie

PREPARATION TIME: 15 MINUTES, PLUS 4 HOURS TO CHILL
COOKING TIME: 55 MINUTES
SERVINGS: 8

1 pound blueberries

1 pound raspberries

1 pound strawberries, hulled and diced

½ cup packed light brown sugar or coconut sugar

2 tablespoons cornstarch

1 tablespoon freshly squeezed lemon juice

½ teaspoon salt

2 disks Basic Gluten-Free Pie Dough

1½ tablespoons coconut oil, melted

1 large egg yolk

1 tablespoon unsweetened dairy-free milk

In a large bowl, stir together the blueberries, raspberries, strawberries, sugar, cornstarch, lemon juice, and salt.

On a lightly floured work surface, roll out one of the dough disks to a 12-inch circle. Transfer to a 9-inch pie pan and press into the bottom and sides. Fill with the berry mixture. Add dots of the oil on top of the berries.

On a lightly floured work surface, roll out the remaining disk to form a 12-inch circle. Place over the filling, trim any excess, and seal and crimp the edges. Cut 3-inch slits on the top of the pie to allow the steam to escape. Refrigerate for 15 minutes.

Preheat the oven to 400°F. Place a baking sheet on a bottom rack to catch any bubbling juices.

In a small bowl, whisk the egg yolk and milk together, and brush over the top of the pie. Place the pie on the center rack of the oven and bake for 20 minutes. Tent it with aluminum foil, allowing air to still flow through, and bake until slightly browned and bubbling in the center, another 35 to 40 minutes. Transfer to a wire rack to cool completely before slicing.

STORAGE: Store covered at room temperature for up to 3 days.

VARIATION: Add 1 teaspoon of ground cardamom to the berries.

249. Marbled Chocolate and Peanut Butter Pie

PREPARATION TIME: 15 MINUTES, PLUS 4 HOURS TO CHILL

COOKING TIME: 55 MINUTES

SERVINGS: 8

1 disk Basic Gluten-Free Pie Dough

2 cups vegan cream cheese, at room temperature

3 large eggs

1 cup natural peanut butter

¼ cup light brown sugar or coconut sugar

3 tablespoons arrowroot

1 tablespoon coconut oil, melted

2 teaspoons vanilla extract

¼ teaspoon salt

½ cup dairy-free chocolate chips

Preheat the oven to 350°F.

On a lightly floured work surface, roll out the dough to a 12-inch circle. Transfer to a 9-inch pie pan and press into the bottom and sides. Crimp the edges, then prick the bottom a few times with a fork. Bake until golden, about 10 minutes. Transfer to a wire rack to cool.

In a large bowl, using an electric mixer on medium speed, beat the cream cheese until smooth and fluffy. Beat in the eggs, peanut butter, sugar, arrowroot, oil, vanilla, and salt until well blended.

In a medium glass bowl, heat the chocolate chips in the microwave for 30 to 60 seconds, just until they start to melt. Stir the chocolate until it is completely melted, then stir in 1 cup of the peanut butter mixture. Pour the remaining peanut butter mixture into the cooled crust. Drop the chocolate mixture by tablespoons over the peanut butter layer, then drag the blade of a knife through the chocolate to swirl it and create a marbled effect.

Bake until the filling is firm around the edges, about 45 minutes. It will be slightly soft in the middle and will continue to set as it cools. Transfer to a wire rack to cool completely. Refrigerate for at least 4 hours before serving.

PREP TIP: When marbling the chocolate, be careful not to overwork it to keep the mixtures from blending together—you want to see the marbling.

STORAGE: Store covered in refrigerator for up to 3 days.

SUBSTITUTIONS: You can swap out the peanut butter for almond butter.

250. Key Lime Pie

PREPARATION TIME: 20 MINUTES, PLUS 2 HOURS TO CHILL
COOKING TIME: 50 MINUTES
SERVINGS: 6 TO 8

1 disk Basic Gluten-Free Pie Dough

2 teaspoons unflavored gelatin

2 tablespoons warm water

½ cup full-fat coconut milk

6 large egg yolks

½ cup plus ⅓ cup granulated sugar, divided

½ cup freshly squeezed key lime juice

Grated zest of 3 key limes (2 teaspoons)

3 large egg whites

½ teaspoon vanilla extract

½ teaspoon cream of tartar

Preheat the oven to 350°F.

On a lightly floured work surface, roll out the dough to a 12-inch circle. Transfer to a 9-inch pie pan and press into the bottom and sides. Crimp the edges, then prick the bottom a few times with a fork. Bake until golden, about 10 minutes. Transfer to a wire rack to cool.

Meanwhile, in a small bowl, mix together the gelatin and water until thickened.

In a large bowl, using an electric mixer on low speed, beat the coconut milk, egg yolks, ½ cup of sugar, the gelatin mixture, lime juice, and lime zest together until combined. Pour into the cooled piecrust.

Bake until a knife inserted in the center comes out clean, 20 to 25 minutes. Transfer to a wire rack to cool.

For the meringue, in a large bowl with an electric mixer on high speed, beat the egg whites, vanilla, and cream of tartar together until foamy. Slowly add the remaining ⅓ cup sugar, about 2 tablespoons at a time, beating until soft peaks form. Spread the meringue over the pie to cover it evenly. Be sure to cover to the crust edges; this will keep the filling from seeping out.

Bake until the meringue peaks are lightly golden brown, 12 to 15 minutes. Transfer the pie to a wire rack to cool completely. Refrigerate for at least 2 hours before serving.

PREP TIP: Make sure not to overmix the meringue; whip only until soft peaks form.

STORAGE: Store covered in the refrigerator for up to 3 days.

VARIATION: Use lemon juice and zest in place of the key lime for lemon meringue pie.

251. Pumpkin Pie

PREPARATION TIME: 20 MINUTES

COOKING TIME: 1 HOUR

SERVINGS: 8

1 disk Basic Gluten-Free Pie Dough

½ cup packed light brown sugar or coconut sugar

1 (15-ouncecan pumpkin purée (not pumpkin pie filling)

¾ cup canned full-fat coconut milk

2 large eggs

1 teaspoon vanilla extract

1 teaspoon ground cinnamon

½ teaspoon ground ginger

¼ teaspoon ground cloves

½ teaspoon salt

1 teaspoon vanilla extract

Preheat the oven to 350°F.

On a lightly floured work surface, roll out the dough to a 12-inch circle. Transfer to a 9-inch pie pan and press into the bottom and sides. Crimp the edges, then prick the bottom a few times with a fork. Bake until golden, about 10 minutes. Transfer to a wire rack to cool.

Increase the oven temperature to 375°F.

In a large bowl, using an electric mixer on medium speed, beat the sugar, pumpkin purée, coconut milk, eggs, vanilla, cinnamon, ginger, cloves, and salt together until well blended. Pour into the cooled piecrust.

Bake until a knife inserted in the center comes out clean, about 50 minutes. Transfer to a wire rack to cool completely.

PREP TIP: Make sure to prick the bottom of the pie crust with a fork or use pie weights over parchment paper. This prevents the crust from puffing up.

STORAGE: Store covered in the refrigerator for up to 5 days.

VARIATION: Add 1½ teaspoons grated orange zest to the pumpkin mixture, and garnish with coconut whipped cream (see hereand orange curls.

252. Blackberry Galette

PREPARATION TIME: 15 MINUTES

COOKING TIME: 50 MINUTES

SERVINGS: 6 TO 8

1 disk Basic Gluten-Free Pie Dough

4 cups blackberries

⅓ cup granulated sugar, plus more for sprinkling

1 tablespoon cornstarch

1 tablespoon freshly squeezed lemon juice

½ teaspoon salt

1 large egg yolk

1 tablespoon unsweetened dairy-free milk

Preheat the oven to 375°F.

On a lightly floured piece of parchment paper, roll out the dough to a 13-inch circle. Transfer the dough on the parchment to a rimmed baking sheet. Refrigerate while preparing the filling.

In a large bowl, carefully toss together the blackberries, sugar, cornstarch, lemon juice, and salt. Remove the crust from the refrigerator. Arrange the fruit in the center, leaving a 1½-inch border all around. Fold the border over the filling, allowing the dough to fall naturally.

In a small bowl, whisk together the egg yolk and milk. Brush over the edges of the galette, and sprinkle lightly with sugar.

Bake until the crust is golden brown and the filling is bubbling, about 50 minutes. Transfer to a wire rack to cool for 15 minutes before slicing.

PREP TIP: Make sure to use a baking sheet with a rim. This prevents any juices from dripping onto the oven floor and burning.

STORAGE: Store covered at room temperature for up to 3 days.

253. Double Chocolate Tart with Raspberries and Coconut Whipped Cream

PREPARATION TIME: 30 MINUTES, PLUS 4 HOURS TO CHILL
COOKING TIME: 20 MINUTES
SERVINGS: 6 TO 8

For the crust

¾ cup raw whole natural almonds

¼ cup pecans

½ teaspoon vanilla extract

1 cup pitted Medjool dates

2 tablespoons unsweetened cocoa powder

2 tablespoons coconut oil, melted

2 tablespoons maple syrup

Pinch salt

1 large egg, beaten

For the filling

¼ cup coconut oil

½ cup dairy-free chocolate chunks

¾ cup packed light brown sugar or coconut sugar

3 tablespoons arrowroot

3 large eggs

2 teaspoons vanilla extract

1 cup coconut whipped cream, plus more for serving (here)

3 cups raspberries

Preheat the oven to 325°F. Lightly coat a 9-inch tart pan with nonstick cooking spray.

For the crust, in a food processor on high, pulse the almonds, pecans, and vanilla together until fine crumbs form. Add the dates, cocoa, oil, maple syrup, and salt and pulse until the mixture sticks together. Press into the bottom and sides of the prepared pan. Bake for 15 minutes. Remove from the oven and brush the bottom with the egg. Return to the oven and bake until slightly browned and firm, about 5 minutes. Transfer to a wire rack to cool.

For the filling, in a small saucepan over medium-low heat, heat the coconut oil and chocolate chunks together, stirring constantly, until melted. Add the sugar and arrowroot and whisk together until smooth and combined.

In a large bowl, using an electric mixer on medium speed, beat the eggs until thick and frothy. Whisk about one-third of the chocolate mixture into the eggs, then whisk the egg mixture into the chocolate mixture in the saucepan. Cook over medium heat for 5 minutes, stirring constantly, until the mixture is thick and glossy and coats the back of a spoon. Remove from the heat and stir in the vanilla. Pour into a bowl and refrigerate until lukewarm, about 30 minutes.

Gently fold 1 cup of whipped cream into the chocolate mixture. Cover the remaining whipped cream and refrigerate until serving. Spread the chocolate filling in the crust. Refrigerate for 4 hours before serving.

Serve with additional whipped cream and raspberries.

PREP TIP: One way to test the doneness of a custard or other thickened sauces is to dip a spoon into the mixture. The sauce is ready when it coats the back of the spoon. Alternately, run a finger through it and if it leaves a clear path, your custard or sauce is properly thickened. If the path disappears quickly, cook for another few minutes and test again.

STORAGE: Store covered in the refrigerator for up to 3 days.

254. Summer Vegetable Tart

PREPARATION TIME: 1 HOUR AND 20 MINUTES

COOKING TIME: 1 HOUR AND 15 MINUTES

SERVINGS: 8

2 pounds cherry tomatoes

1 tablespoon balsamic vinegar, plus extra for garnish

1 small zucchini, thinly sliced (about 2 cups)

1 small yellow squash, thinly sliced (about 2 cups)

3 teaspoons salt, divided

1 small red onion, thinly sliced

1 tablespoon extra-virgin olive oil

Freshly ground black pepper

1 disk Basic Gluten-Free Pie Dough

1 large egg, beaten

8 ounces vegan cream cheese

2 garlic cloves, minced

1 tablespoon chopped fresh basil, plus more for garnish

1 teaspoon chopped fresh thyme (use lemon thyme if possible)

Preheat the oven to 400°F. Place a baking sheet on the bottom rack to catch any drippings.

Place the tomatoes on a roasting pan and drizzle with the vinegar. Roast until they are soft and lightly charred, about 45 minutes.

Meanwhile, in a colander, toss the zucchini and squash with 2 teaspoons of salt. Let drain over the sink for 30 minutes. Gently squeeze out any extra water and transfer to a medium bowl. Add the onion and oil, season with pepper to taste, and toss to combine and coat with the oil.

On a floured work surface, roll out the dough to an 11-inch circle. Transfer to a 9-inch pie pan and press into the bottom and sides. Trim the edges, then prick the bottom a few times with a fork. Freeze for 10 minutes.

Bake the crust for 20 minutes. Remove from the oven and brush with the beaten egg. Return to the oven and bake until golden, about 10 minutes. Let cool for 10 minutes.

In a small bowl, beat the cream cheese, garlic, basil, and thyme together until well blended. Spread over the bottom of the cooled tart. Arrange the zucchini and squash on top, then top the squash with the roasted tomatoes.

Bake until the top starts to brown and most of the liquid has evaporated, 35 to 45 minutes. Season with salt and pepper to taste. Garnish with fresh basil and a drizzle of balsamic vinegar.

PREP TIPS:

Make sure to squeeze as much liquid as possible from the squash and zucchini to prevent a soggy tart.

Brushing egg onto the crust helps bind it and allows it to crisp.

STORAGE: Store covered in the refrigerator for up to 3 days or in a zip-top plastic bag in the freezer for up to 1 month.

255. Bacon, Mushroom, and Thyme Quiche

PREPARATION TIME: 20 MINUTES

COOKING TIME: 45 MINUTES

SERVINGS: 6

1 tablespoon extra-virgin olive oil

2 cups sliced mushrooms

2 teaspoons chopped fresh thyme

1 disk Basic Gluten-Free Pie Dough

4 slices turkey bacon or regular bacon

5 large eggs

1 cup plain dairy-free yogurt

¼ teaspoon salt

⅛ teaspoon freshly ground black pepper

Pinch ground nutmeg

In a medium nonstick skillet over medium-high heat, heat the oil. Then add the mushrooms and cook, stirring a few times, until tender and the water has evaporated, about 5 minutes. Add the thyme and toss to coat. Remove from the heat.

Preheat the oven to 400°F.

On a lightly floured work surface, roll out the dough to an 11-inch circle. Transfer to a 9-inch tart pan and press into the bottom and sides. Trim the edges, then prick the bottom a few times with a fork. Bake until golden, about 10 minutes. Transfer to a wire rack to cool.

In a small skillet over medium-high heat, cook the bacon, turning, until crisp, about 4 minutes. Place between two paper towels to remove extra oil. Set aside.

In a large bowl, whisk together the eggs, yogurt, salt, pepper, and nutmeg.

Crumble the bacon over the baked piecrust. Top with the mushrooms, then the egg mixture.

Bake until a knife inserted in the center comes out clean, 30 to 35 minutes. If the piecrust starts to burn on the edges, tent with aluminum foil and continue baking.

Remove from the oven and serve.

REHEATING TIP: If the quiche has been made in advance, cover it with foil and reheat in the oven at 325°F until heated through.

STORAGE: Store covered in the refrigerator for up to 3 days.

256. Spinach and Sun-Dried Tomato Potato-Crusted Quiche

PREPARATION TIME: 25 MINUTES

COOKING TIME: 1 HOUR

SERVINGS: 4 TO 6

2 or 3 large Yukon Gold potatoes, thinly sliced

½ cup drained and chopped oil-packed sun-dried tomatoes, plus 3 tablespoons reserved oil, divided

5 large eggs

1½ cups plain dairy-free yogurt

¼ cup arrowroot

½ teaspoon salt

¼ teaspoon freshly ground black pepper

1 tablespoon chopped fresh basil

Pinch ground nutmeg

⅓ cup chopped scallions (green parts only)

1 cup chopped spinach

Preheat the oven to 450°F. Place a baking sheet on the bottom rack to catch any drippings. Lightly coat a 9-inch pie pan with nonstick cooking spray.

Line the bottom and sides of the pan with the potato slices. Drizzle with 2 tablespoons of reserved oil from the tomatoes. Bake until slightly browned, about 10 minutes. Transfer to a wire rack to cool.

Reduce the oven temperature to 350°F.

In a large bowl, whisk together the eggs, yogurt, arrowroot, salt, pepper, basil, and nutmeg. Stir in the scallions, tomatoes, and remaining 1 tablespoon of reserved oil.

Scatter the spinach over the potato slices. Top with the egg mixture.

Bake until a knife inserted in the center comes out clean, 50 to 60 minutes. Let cool on a wire rack for 20 minutes before slicing.

PREP TIP: Make sure the potato slices overlap slightly to fully cover the bottom of the pie pan.

STORAGE: Store covered in the refrigerator for up to 3 days.

SUBSTITUTIONS: Substitute kale for the spinach. For a little extra sweetness, use sweet potatoes instead of the Yukon potatoes.

257. Chicken-Mushroom Pot Pie

PREPARATION TIME: 30 MINUTES
COOKING TIME: 45 MINUTES
SERVINGS: 8

1 tablespoon extra-virgin olive oil

2 cups chopped carrots

1 cup chopped scallions (green and white parts)

1 cup sliced mushrooms

¾ cup thinly sliced celery

1 tablespoon chopped fresh rosemary

1 teaspoon poultry seasoning

1 cup unsweetened dairy-free milk

1½ cups chicken broth

4 tablespoons vegan butter

⅓ cup cornstarch

¾ teaspoon salt

¼ teaspoon freshly ground pepper

2 chicken breasts, cooked and diced

1 cup frozen peas

¼ cup chopped fresh parsley

1 disk Basic Gluten-Free Pie Dough

Pinch granulated sugar

Preheat the oven to 350°F.

In a medium saucepan, heat the oil over medium-high heat, Add the carrots, scallions, mushrooms, and celery and cook, stirring, until the vegetables are tender, about 10 minutes. Stir in the rosemary and poultry seasoning. Transfer to a large bowl.

In the same saucepan, whisk together the milk, broth, butter, arrowroot, salt, and pepper. Over medium heat, bring to a simmer and cook, whisking, until it starts to thicken, about 10 minutes. Carefully add to the bowl with the vegetables. Stir the chicken, peas, and parsley into the bowl with the sauce. Pour into a 9-inch pie pan.

On a lightly floured work surface, roll out the dough to a 10-inch circle. Place over the chicken mixture and crimp the edges. Cut a few slashes in the crust to allow steam to escape.

Bake until the crust is golden brown and the filling is bubbly, about 40 to 45 minutes. Let cool for 10 minutes before serving.

PREP TIP: If the dough becomes too warm to handle, spread it on a floured sheet of parchment paper, transfer to a baking pan, and freeze for 5 to 10 minutes.

STORAGE: Store covered in the refrigerator for up to 3 days.

258. Warm Peach Cobbler

PREPARATION TIME: 20 MINUTES

COOKING TIME: 25 MINUTES

SERVINGS: 6 TO 8

For the filling

8 large ripe peaches, pitted and cut into small chunks

¼ cup maple syrup

2½ tablespoons arrowroot or cornstarch

2 tablespoons freshly squeezed lemon juice

1 teaspoon ground nutmeg

1 teaspoon ground cinnamon

1 teaspoon vanilla extract

⅓ cup packed light brown sugar or coconut sugar

For the topping

1 cup plus 1 tablespoon Basic Gluten-Free Flour Blend or store-bought equivalent

½ cup granulated sugar, divided

1 tablespoon psyllium husk

1¼ teaspoons baking powder

½ teaspoon xanthan gum

½ teaspoon salt

¼ teaspoon baking soda

6 tablespoons coconut oil, chilled until very solid

⅓ cup vanilla dairy-free yogurt

2 tablespoons water

1 large egg white, beaten

Preheat the oven to 400°F. Lightly coat a 9-inch square baking pan with nonstick cooking spray.

For the filling, in a large bowl, stir together the peaches, maple syrup, arrowroot, lemon juice, nutmeg, cinnamon, and vanilla. Place in the prepared pan. Sprinkle with the sugar. Bake for 10 minutes.

For the topping, in a large bowl, whisk together the flour blend, ¼ cup of the sugar, the psyllium husk, baking powder, xanthan gum, salt, and baking soda. Using a pastry blender or two knives, cut in the oil until crumbly with pea-size chunks. With a fork, stir in the yogurt and water just until moist and somewhat sticky.

Carefully spoon the topping over the peaches. Cover as evenly as possible, leaving just a few open spots. Brush the top with the egg white and sprinkle with the remaining ¼ cup of sugar.

Bake until the fruit is bubbling and a toothpick inserted in the center comes out clean, 10 to 15 minutes. Transfer to a wire rack to cool.

STORAGE: Store covered in the refrigerator for up to 3 days.

VARIATION: Turn this into plum or nectarine cobbler using the same amount of fruit as the peaches.

259. Apple-Cranberry Crumble

PREPARATION TIME: 15 MINUTES

COOKING TIME: 45 MINUTES

SERVINGS: 8 TO 10

3 medium Pink Lady apples, cored, peeled, and finely chopped

2 cups fresh or frozen cranberries

1 tablespoon granulated sugar

1 teaspoon ground cinnamon

1½ cups certified gluten-free rolled oats

¼ cup Basic Gluten-Free Flour Blend or store-bought equivalent

½ cup packed light brown sugar or coconut sugar

½ cup chopped walnuts or pecans

½ cup maple syrup or honey

½ cup coconut oil, melted

Pinch salt

Preheat the oven to 350°F. Lightly coat a 9-inch square baking pan with nonstick cooking spray.

In a large bowl, stir together the apples, cranberries, granulated sugar, and cinnamon until well blended. Pour into the prepared pan.

In a food processor, pulse the oats, flour blend, brown sugar, walnuts, maple syrup, oil, and salt one or two times to mix gently, but do not process the oats too finely. Crumble the oat mixture evenly over the apples.

Bake until the topping starts to brown and the fruit bubbles, 40 to 45 minutes. Serve slightly warm or chilled.

STORAGE: Store covered at room temperature for up to 3 days.

SUBSTITUTIONS: You can turn this into an apple crumble by using five to six apples and omitting the cranberries.

260. Coconut-Raisin Baked Rice Pudding

PREPARATION TIME: 15 MINUTES, PLUS 2 HOURS TO CHILL
COOKING TIME: 50 MINUTES
SERVINGS: 6 TO 8

3 cups cooked rice, cooled

½ cup raisins

2 (15-ouncecans full-fat coconut milk

¾ cup granulated sugar

3 large eggs

½ cup unsweetened shredded coconut

2 teaspoons vanilla extract

1½ teaspoons ground cinnamon

1 teaspoon cornstarch

Grated zest from 1 small lemon (½ teaspoon)

¼ teaspoon ground nutmeg

¼ teaspoon salt

Place a large roasting pan filled halfway with water in the oven. Preheat the oven to 350°F. Lightly coat a 9-inch square baking pan with nonstick cooking spray.

Sprinkle the cooked rice evenly in the prepared pan. Top with the raisins.

In a large bowl, whisk the coconut milk, sugar, eggs, coconut, vanilla, cinnamon, cornstarch, lemon zest, nutmeg, and salt together. Pour over the rice and raisins.

Carefully place the baking pan in the roasting pan in the oven; the water should reach halfway up the sides of the baking pan. Bake until slightly browned and a knife inserted in the center comes out clean, 40 to 50 minutes.

Remove from the water bath and place the square pan on a wire rack to cool. Cover and refrigerate for at least 2 hours before serving.

261. Sweet Breads

PREPARATION TIME: 15 minutes, plus 1 hour to prepare the sponge and 45 minutes to rise
COOKING TIME: 40 minutes
SERVINGS: 1 LOAF
TOOLS
Plastic wrap
6-by-10-inch baking dish
Parchment paper
½ cup candied citrus peel
½ cup raisins or dried cranberries
½ cup brandy
1 cup brown rice flour
¼ cup plus 2 tablespoons potato starch
2 tablespoons tapioca starch
½ cup whole milk or nondairy milk, warmed to 110°F
1 (¼-ouncepacket active dry yeast
¾ teaspoon xanthan gum
½ tablespoon sugar
½ teaspoon sea salt
½ teaspoon ground cinnamon
1 egg, at room temperature
2½ tablespoons butter or nondairy butter, at room temperature
Zest of 1 lemon
Zest of 1 orange
2 ounces marzipan
Vegetable oil, for brushing
Powdered sugar

Combine the candied citrus peel, raisins, and brandy in a nonreactive dish to soak. Set aside.

In a large bowl, sift together the brown rice flour, potato starch, and tapioca starch.

To make the sponge, transfer ½ cup of the flour mixture to a large glass measuring cup or another nonreactive dish. Add the warmed milk and yeast. Whisk to blend. Cover the sponge with plastic wrap and set aside for 1 hour.

To the large bowl with the remaining flour mixture, add the xanthan gum, sugar, salt, and cinnamon.

Add the sponge, egg, butter, lemon zest, and orange zest. Beat for 30 seconds. Scrape down the sides of the bowl, and mix for 3 minutes.

Line a 6-by-10-inch baking dish with parchment paper.

Place slightly more than half of the dough into the dish and spread it to the edges.

Cut the marzipan into rectangles and lay them down the center of the dough. The row of marzipan should be about 3 inches wide by 8 inches long.

Top the marzipan with the remaining bread dough, mounding it up in the center to form a tall log shape, though it will not be perfectly round.

Allow to rise at room temperature for about 45 minutes. It will rise by about 50 percent but not double in size.

1Preheat the oven to 350°F. Bake for 40 minutes until the bread is deeply browned. It should register 190°F in the center of the loaf.

1Immediately brush the bread with oil, and use a fine-mesh sieve to sift powdered sugar over the top. Wait 5 minutes and repeat the application of powdered sugar.

INGREDIENT TIP: To make your own candied citrus peel, place 1 cup lemon, orange, and grapefruit peel cut into ¼-inch-wide slices into a pot of boiling water. Cook for 10 minutes, then drain. Bring 1 cup sugar and 1 cup water to a simmer, stirring to dissolve the sugar. Cook the citrus peel in the sugar water for 10 more minutes. Strain, reserving the cooking liquid, and transfer the citrus peel to a mesh cooling rack. You can use the reserved liquid to add a hint of sweetness to salad dressings or sparkling water. You can also use it to make your own glühwein, a German mulled wine—it works well because you don't have to cook the wine to dissolve the sugar.

262. apple kuchen

PREPARATION TIME: 15 minutes, plus 45 minutes to rise
COOKING TIME: 25 minutes

SERVINGS: 8

TOOLS

Springform pan

For the glaze

½ cup powdered sugar

1 tablespoon milk or nondairy milk

For the cake

5 tablespoons butter or nondairy butter, at room temperature, divided

2 cups plus 1 tablespoon White Bread Flour Blend, divided

½ cup milk or nondairy milk, warmed to 110°F

1 (¼-ouncepacket active dry yeast

3 tablespoons sugar

1 teaspoon xanthan gum

¾ teaspoon sea salt

3 eggs, at room temperature, divided

1 teaspoon vanilla extract

2 tablespoons heavy cream or nondairy cream

2 apples, peeled, cored, and finely diced

2 tablespoons toasted sliced almonds

To make the glaze

In a small bowl, whisk together the powdered sugar and milk. Set aside.

To make the cake

Coat the interior of a springform pan with 1 tablespoon of butter, and dust with 1 tablespoon of flour blend. Set aside.

In a small bowl, mix together ¼ cup of flour blend with the warm milk and yeast.

In a large bowl, mix together the remaining 1¾ cups of flour blend, sugar, xanthan gum, and salt.

Add the yeast-milk mixture to the bowl, along with the remaining 4 tablespoons of butter, 2 eggs, and vanilla. Mix for 15 seconds. Scrape down the sides of the bowl with a spatula. Mix for an additional 3 minutes.

Transfer the dough to the prepared pan. Allow the dough to rise for 45 minutes, until puffy. Meanwhile, preheat the oven to 375°F.

In a small bowl, whisk the cream and the remaining egg until thoroughly blended. Pour the mixture over the risen dough. Gently sprinkle the apples and almonds on top.

Bake for 22 to 25 minutes, until the top is golden brown and the center is set.

Drizzle the glaze over the cooked apple kuchen. Allow to rest for at least 30 minutes before serving.

INGREDIENT TIP: To reduce the sugar, simply omit the powdered sugar glaze and add 1 tablespoon brown sugar to the cream-egg mixture.

263. brioche

PREPARATION TIME: 10 minutes, plus 1 hour to prepare the sponge
COOKING TIME: 20 minutes
SERVINGS: 6 (4-INCHBRIOCHE
TOOLS
6 brioche molds
Plastic wrap
Rimmed baking sheet
10 tablespoons (1¼ sticksbutter or nondairy butter, at room temperature, divided
2 cups plus 2 tablespoons White Bread Flour Blend, divided
3 tablespoons sugar, divided
½ cup milk or nondairy milk, warmed to 110°F
1 (¼-ouncepacket active dry yeast
1 teaspoon xanthan gum
¾ teaspoon sea salt
3 eggs, at room temperature

Coat the insides of the brioche molds with 2 tablespoons of butter and sprinkle with 2 tablespoons of flour blend. Set aside.

Place ½ cup of flour blend in a large glass measuring cup or another nonreactive dish. Add 1 tablespoon of sugar, warmed milk, and yeast, and whisk to blend. Cover with plastic wrap and set aside for 1 hour to form a sponge.

In a large bowl, combine the remaining 1½ cups of flour blend, the remaining 2 tablespoons of sugar, xanthan gum, and salt. Add the sponge, the remaining 8 tablespoons of butter, and eggs. Mix for 15 seconds. Scrape down the sides of the bowl. Mix for 3 additional minutes.

Divide the dough between the molds. Set the molds on a rimmed baking sheet and allow the dough to rise for 1 hour.

Preheat the oven to 350°F.

Bake the brioche for 17 to 19 minutes, until golden brown and puffy.

Allow to rest for 15 minutes before serving.

INGREDIENT TIP: To quickly warm eggs to room temperature, place them in a bowl of warm (but not hotwater for 15 minutes.

264. croissants

PREPARATION TIME: 1 hour plus 11 hours to chill
COOKING TIME: 45 minutes
SERVINGS: 20 CROISSANTS
TOOLS
Stand mixer (optional)
Parchment paper
Plastic wrap
Baking dish
2 baking sheets
For the butter block
2 tablespoons White Bread Flour Blend
1 cup (2 sticksunsalted butter, barely softened (see Ingredient tip)
For the croissants
3⅓ cups White Bread Flour Blend, plus more for dusting
2 tablespoons sugar
1 (¼-ouncepacket active dry yeast
2 teaspoons xanthan gum
1½ teaspoons sea salt
1 tablespoon butter, melted, plus more for greasing
1¼ cups 2 percent milk, warmed to 110°F
1 egg
1 tablespoon water
To make the butter block

In a large bowl or the bowl of a stand mixer fitted with the paddle attachment, combine the flour blend and butter. Mix until well blended, about 2 minutes, scraping the butter away from the paddle (if usingas needed.

Place the butter block onto a large sheet of parchment paper, and shape into a rectangle about 5 inches by 7 inches. Fold the parchment over it to seal. Place in the refrigerator for 1 hour, or until firm but pliable enough to make an indentation by pressing with your fingertip.

To make the croissants

Clean the bowl, then combine the flour blend, sugar, yeast, xanthan gum, and salt. Add the melted butter and warm milk, and mix for 15 seconds by hand or with the paddle attachment. Scrape down the sides of the bowl. Mix for 3 additional minutes.

Lightly grease another large bowl with butter, and transfer the dough into it. Place the bowl in the refrigerator for 2 hours.

Remove the dough and the butter block from the refrigerator.

Lightly dust a large sheet of parchment paper with flour blend. Roll the dough into a rectangle about 8 inches by 11 inches, with the shorter side facing you. Place the butter block onto the dough along the side closest to you (figure A). (The 7-inch side of the butter block should be next to the 8-inch side of the dough.Fold the remaining half of the dough over the butter block (figure B), and gently seal it along the edges (figure C).

Dust the dough with flour blend to prevent the rolling pin from sticking.

Roll the dough with the butter block inside it, until it is again about 8 inches by 11 inches.

Fold the dough into thirds, as if folding a business letter.

Again, roll the dough out until it is roughly 8 inches by 11 inches.

Again, fold the dough as if folding a business letter. Wrap the dough tightly in plastic wrap and place in the refrigerator for 1 hour 30 minutes.

1Repeat steps 3 through 9, but refrigerate the dough overnight.

1Preheat the oven to 300°F for 1 minute until it reaches 80°F. Turn off the oven. Place a baking dish containing 2 cups of hot water on the bottom rack. Line 2 baking sheets with parchment paper and set aside.

1Remove the dough from the refrigerator, divide it into 2 portions, and return 1 portion, wrapped tightly in plastic wrap, to the refrigerator.

1Place a large, clean sheet of parchment paper on the work surface. Dust it lightly with flour blend to prevent the croissant dough from sticking.

1Roll the dough out into a large rectangle until it is less than ¼ inch thick. Make sure it does not stick to the parchment paper by turning the dough, or even flipping it once, before it is fully rolled out.

Divide the rectangle into 2 narrow rectangles. Use a sharp knife or pizza wheel to cut these into triangles (figure D).

1One at a time, carefully lift each triangle from the parchment and roll it loosely, starting at the bottom and rolling toward the point. Gently curve the ends of the roll into a crescent shape and place the dough onto a prepared baking sheet (figure E). The tip of the dough (what was once the top of the triangleshould fold over the top of the croissant down toward the baking sheet but should not be tucked under.

Repeat with the remaining dough to fill 1 baking sheet. Place in the warmed oven to rise for 2 hours.

Remove the second block of dough from the refrigerator and repeat steps 11 through 17.

Remove both baking sheets from the oven and set them on the counter. Remove the baking dish with the steaming water.

Preheat the oven to 400°F.

In a small bowl, whisk the egg and water. Very gently brush the tops of the croissants with the egg wash. Place the first baking sheet on the middle rack in the oven and bake for 22 minutes, until the croissants are puffy and golden brown. Repeat with the second baking sheet.

Allow to cool completely before enjoying.

BAKING TIP: Avoid setting the baking sheets on top of the oven while it preheats. This will cause them to overproof.

INGREDIENT TIP: Allow cold butter to sit on the countertop for up to 30 minutes to let it soften slightly but not come up to room temperature.

Figure A

Figure B

Figure C

Figure D

Figure E

265. almond croissants

PREPARATION TIME: 1 hour plus 11 hours to chill
COOKING TIME: 45 minutes
SERVINGS: 20 CROISSANTS
TOOLS
Stand mixer (optional)
Parchment paper
Plastic wrap
Baking dish
2 baking sheets
For the butter block
2 tablespoons White Bread Flour Blend
1 cup (2 sticksunsalted butter, barely softened (see Ingredient tip)
For the croissants
3⅓ cups White Bread Flour
Blend (here), plus more for dusting
2 tablespoons granulated sugar
1 (¼-ouncepacket active dry yeast
2 teaspoons xanthan gum
1½ teaspoons sea salt
1 tablespoon butter, melted, plus more for greasing
1¼ cups 2 percent milk, warmed to 110°F
8 ounces marzipan
1 egg
1 tablespoon water
½ cup thinly sliced toasted almonds
4 tablespoons powdered sugar
To make the butter block

In a large bowl or the bowl of a stand mixer fitted with the paddle attachment, combine the flour blend and butter. Mix until well blended, about 2 minutes, scraping the butter away from the paddle, if using, a few times as needed.

Place the butter block onto a large sheet of parchment paper and shape into a rectangle about 5 inches by 7 inches. Fold the parchment over it to seal.

Place in the refrigerator for 1 hour, or until firm but pliable enough to make an indentation by pressing with your fingertip.

To make the croissants

Clean the bowl, then combine the flour blend, sugar, yeast, xanthan gum, and salt. Add the melted butter and warm milk, and mix for 15 seconds using the paddle attachment or by hand. Scrape down the sides of the bowl. Mix for 3 additional minutes.

Lightly grease another large bowl with butter, and transfer the dough into it. Place the bowl in the refrigerator for 2 hours.

Remove the dough and the butter block from the refrigerator.

Lightly dust a large sheet of parchment paper with flour blend. Roll the dough into a rectangle about 8 inches by 11 inches, with the shorter side facing you. Place the butter block onto the dough along the side closest to you. (The 7-inch side of the butter block should be next to the 8-inch side of the dough.Fold the remaining half of the dough over the butter block and gently seal it along the edges.

Dust the dough with flour to prevent the rolling pin from sticking.

Roll the dough with the butter block inside it, until it is again about 8 inches by 11 inches.

Fold the dough into thirds as if folding a business letter.

Again, roll the dough out until it is roughly 8 inches by 11 inches.

Again, fold the dough as if folding a business letter. Wrap the dough tightly in plastic wrap and place in the refrigerator for 1 hour 30 minutes.

1Repeat steps 3 through 9, but refrigerate the dough overnight.

1Preheat the oven to 300°F for 1 minute until it reaches a temperature of 80°F. Turn off the oven. Place a baking dish containing 2 cups of hot water on the bottom rack of the oven. Line 2 baking sheets with parchment paper and set aside.

1Remove the dough from the refrigerator, divide it into 2 portions, and return 1 portion, wrapped tightly in plastic wrap, to the refrigerator.Place a large, clean sheet of parchment paper on the work surface. Dust it lightly with flour blend to prevent the croissant dough from sticking.

Roll the dough out into a large rectangle, until it is less than ¼ inch thick. Make sure it does not stick to the parchment paper by turning the dough, or even flipping it once, before it is fully rolled out.

Divide the rectangle into 2 narrow rectangles. Cut these into triangles using a sharp knife or a pizza wheel.

One at a time, carefully lift each triangle from the parchment. Place about 2 teaspoons of marzipan onto the bottom of the triangle, and roll it loosely, starting at the bottom and rolling toward the point. Gently curve the ends of the roll into a crescent shape, and place the dough onto a prepared baking sheet. The point of the dough should fold over the top of the croissant down toward the baking sheet, but should not be tucked under.

Repeat with the remaining dough to fill 1 baking sheet. Place in the warmed oven to rise for 2 hours.

Remove the second block of dough from the refrigerator, and repeat steps 11 through 17.

Remove both baking sheets from the oven and set them on the counter. Remove the baking dish with the steaming water.

Preheat the oven to 400°F.

In a small bowl, whisk together the egg and water. Very gently brush the tops of the croissants with the egg wash, and sprinkle with the almonds. Place the first baking sheet on the middle rack in the oven and bake for 22 minutes, until the croissants are puffy and golden brown. Immediately sift 1 tablespoon of powdered sugar over the top of all of the croissants.

Repeat step 21 with the second baking sheet.

Allow to cool completely before enjoying.

INGREDIENT TIP: Marzipan is made from ground blanched almonds and sugar. It can be purchased in a sealed container in the baking aisle.

INGREDIENT TIP: Allow cold butter to sit on the countertop for up to 30 minutes to let it soften slightly but not come up to room temperature.

266. pain au chocolat

PREPARATION TIME: 1 hour plus 11 hours to chill
COOKING TIME: 45 minutes
SERVINGS: 20 PASTRIES
TOOLS
Stand mixer (optional)

Parchment paper

Plastic wrap

Baking dish

2 baking sheets

For the butter block

2 tablespoons White Bread Flour Blend

1 cup (2 sticksunsalted butter, barely softened (see Ingredient tip)

For the pastries

3⅓ cups White Bread Flour Blend, plus more for dusting

2 tablespoons sugar

1 (¼-ouncepacket active dry yeast

2 teaspoons xanthan gum

1½ teaspoons sea salt

1 tablespoon butter, melted, plus more (not meltedfor greasing

1¼ cups 2 percent milk, warmed to 110°F

1½ cups 60 percent cacao chocolate chips

1 egg

1 tablespoon water

To make the butter block

In a large bowl or the bowl of a stand mixer fitted with the paddle attachment, combine the flour blend and butter. Mix until well blended, about 2 minutes, scraping the butter away from the paddle, if using, as needed.

Place the butter block onto a large sheet of parchment paper and shape into a rectangle about 5 inches by 7 inches. Fold the parchment over it to seal. Place in the refrigerator for 1 hour, or until firm but pliable enough to make an indentation by pressing with your fingertip.

To make the pastries

Clean the bowl, then mix together the flour blend, sugar, yeast, xanthan gum, and salt. Add the melted butter and warm milk, and mix for 15 seconds using the paddle attachment or by hand. Scrape down the sides of the bowl. Mix for 3 additional minutes.

Lightly grease another large bowl with butter, and transfer the dough into it. Place the bowl in the refrigerator for 2 hours.

Remove the dough and the butter block from the refrigerator.

Lightly dust a large sheet of parchment paper with flour blend. Roll the dough into a rectangle about 8 inches by 11 inches, with the shorter side facing you. Place the butter block onto the dough along the side closest to you. (The 7-inch side of the butter block should be next to the 8-inch side of the dough.Fold the remaining half of the dough over the butter block and gently seal it along the edges.

Dust the dough with flour to prevent the rolling pin from sticking.

Roll the dough with the butter block inside it, until it is again about 8 inches by 11 inches.

Fold the dough into thirds as if folding a business letter.

Again, roll the dough out until it is roughly 8 inches by 11 inches.

Again, fold the dough as if folding a business letter. Wrap the dough tightly in plastic wrap, and place in the refrigerator for 1 hour 30 minutes.

1Repeat steps 3 through 9, but refrigerate the dough overnight.

1Preheat the oven to 300°F for 1 minute until it reaches 80°F. Turn off the oven. Place a baking dish containing 2 cups of hot water on the bottom rack of the oven. Line 2 baking sheets with parchment paper and set aside.

1Remove the dough from the refrigerator, divide it into 2 portions, and return 1 portion, wrapped tightly in plastic wrap, to the refrigerator.

1Place a large, clean sheet of parchment paper onto the work surface. Dust it lightly with flour blend to prevent the dough from sticking.

1Roll the dough out into a large rectangle until it is less than ¼ inch thick. Make sure it does not stick to the parchment paper by turning the dough, or even flipping it once, before it is fully rolled out.

1Divide the rectangle into 2 narrow rectangles. Using a sharp knife or pizza wheel, cut these into a total of 10 rectangles.

1Place 1 generous tablespoon of chocolate chips onto each rectangle and fold the dough tightly over the chocolate. Place the pastries onto 1 prepared baking sheet, and place in the warmed oven to rise for 2 hours.

1Remove the second block of dough from the refrigerator, and repeat steps 11 through 16.

1Remove both baking sheets from the oven and set them on the counter. Remove the baking dish with the steaming water.

1Preheat the oven to 400°F.

2In a small bowl, whisk together the egg and water. Very gently brush the tops of the pastries with the egg wash. Place the first baking sheet onto the middle rack in the oven and bake for 15 to 18 minutes, until the pastries are puffy and golden brown. Repeat with the second baking sheet.

2Allow to cool completely before enjoying.

BAKING TIP: If you are having trouble sealing the pastries without smashing the dough, brush them gently with the egg wash before folding.

INGREDIENT TIP: Allow cold butter to sit on the countertop for up to 30 minutes to let it soften slightly but not come up to room temperature.

VARIATION TIP: This dough is also excellent for making savory pastries, such as salmon en croute or any other recipe requiring a puff pastry.

267. cinnamon rolls

PREPARATION TIME: 15 minutes, plus 45 minutes to 1 hour to rise
COOKING TIME: 25 minutes
SERVINGS: 8 ROLLS
TOOLS
8-inch pie plate or cake pan
Parchment paper
For the filling
¼ cup brown sugar
1 teaspoon ground cinnamon
For the glaze
½ cup powdered sugar
1 tablespoon milk or nondairy milk
For the rolls
2 cups White Bread Flour Blend (here), divided, plus more for dusting
½ cup milk or nondairy milk, warmed to 110°F
1 (¼-ouncepacket active dry yeast
¼ cup sugar
1 teaspoon xanthan gum
¾ teaspoon sea salt
3 tablespoons butter or nondairy butter, at room temperature, plus
1 tablespoon butter or nondairy butter, melted
2 eggs, at room temperature
To make the filling
In a small bowl, mix together the brown sugar and cinnamon. Set aside.
To make the glaze
In another small bowl, whisk together the powdered sugar and milk. Set aside.
To make the rolls
Line the interior of an 8-inch pie plate or cake pan with parchment paper. Set aside.
In a nonreactive dish, combine ¼ cup of flour blend with the warm milk and yeast.
In a large bowl, mix the remaining 1¾ cups flour blend, sugar, xanthan gum, and salt.

Add the yeast-milk mixture to the bowl along with the 3 tablespoons of butter and eggs. Mix for 15 seconds. Scrape down the sides of the bowl with a spatula. Mix for 3 additional minutes.

Line a clean work surface with parchment paper. Sprinkle generously with additional flour blend.

Transfer the dough from the mixer to the prepared work surface and spread into a rectangle about 6 inches by 10 inches; the long edge should be nearest to you.

Brush the dough with the melted butter. Sprinkle the filling over the dough.

Lift one end of the parchment paper to help you roll the dough from one of the short ends to the other (across the work surface from left to right). It should easily release from the floured parchment. If parts of it stick, use a sharp knife to "peel" it from the parchment.

Roll the dough into the shape of a log. It will be somewhat flat. Use a clean knife to cut the dough into 2-inch rolls. Using the knife, transfer each roll into the prepared pan, nudging the dough into the desired round shape. Repeat with the remaining dough, scraping excess dough from the knife as needed.

1Allow the dough to rise for 45 minutes to 1 hour, until very puffy. Preheat the oven to 375°F.

1Bake for 20 to 22 minutes, until the tops are golden brown and the center is still somewhat soft.

1Drizzle the glaze over the baked cinnamon rolls. Allow to rest for 10 to 15 minutes before serving.

BAKING TIP: A slower rise is better for these cinnamon rolls, so let them rise on the countertop instead of in a warmed oven, unless the ambient temperature in your home is well below 70°F.

268. popovers

PREPARATION TIME: 10 minutes
COOKING TIME: 25 minutes

SERVINGS: 12 POPOVERS

TOOLS

12-cup popover pan or muffin tin (see Baking tip)

4 tablespoons butter or nondairy butter, melted, divided

1½ cups Multigrain Flour Blend

1 tablespoon sugar

¼ teaspoon xanthan gum

⅛ teaspoon sea salt

3 eggs, at room temperature

1½ cups milk or nondairy milk, at room temperature

Preheat the oven to 425°F. Coat the interiors of the popover cups with 2 tablespoons of butter.

In a large bowl, whisk the flour blend, sugar, xanthan gum, and salt. Add the remaining 2 tablespoons of butter, eggs, and milk, and whisk until no lumps remain.

When the oven is preheated, place the prepared pan into it for 2 minutes. Remove the pan from the oven, and pour the mixture into the heated pan so each cup is about half full.

Bake for 25 minutes, until the popovers are gorgeously risen and browned.

BAKING TIP: A muffin tin is the most likely substitute for a proper popover pan, but it is not quite as deep and the walls of the cups are slanted, which affects the result. If you use a muffin tin, reduce the volume of ingredients by roughly one-third: Use 3 tablespoons butter, 1 cup flour blend, 2 teaspoons sugar, scant ¼ teaspoon xanthan gum, scant ⅛ teaspoon salt, 2 eggs, and 1 cup milk.

TROUBLESHOOTING TIP: Like other egg-leavened dishes, popovers require that you don't open the oven during baking.

269. Trampoline Cake

Preparation time: 25 minutes

Cooking time: 1 hour

Servings: 12

Nutrition:

Carbohydrates – 25.2 g

Fat – 1.7 g

Protein – 2.4 g

Calories – 126

Ingredients:

7 medium eggs, separated, at room temperature (70°F

½ cup orange juice

1 tsp vanilla flavoring or extract

½ tsp cream of tartar

1½ cups sugar

½ cup rice flour

½ cup tapioca flour

1 tsp baking powder

1 tsp xanthan gum

1½ tsp salt

Directions:

Grease a 9-inch tube pan or an 11 x 7-inch cake pan; sprinkle with rice flour.

Beat egg whites until foamy but not overly stiff.

Fold in cream of tartar to beaten whites.

Beat egg yolks in separate bowl.

Whisk yolks and sugar together until they form a "ribbon" as the mixture flows off the whisk.

Whisk orange juice and vanilla gradually into beaten yolks.

Add flours, baking powder, xanthan gum, and salt to yolk mixture. Blend.

Fold beaten egg whites into yolks.

Bake at 325°F for 30 minutes.

Reset oven temperature to 350°F. Bake for 30 minutes longer.

270. Zucchini Cake

Preparation time: 15 minutes

Cooking time: 60 minutes

Servings: 20

Nutrition:

Carbohydrates – 31.1 g

Fat – 43.4 g

Protein – 18.2 g

Calories – 588

Ingredients:

6 cups almond meal flour

4 tsp cinnamon

1 tsp baking soda

2 tsp baking powder

½ cup plain nuts, chopped

3 tsp xanthan gum

½ tsp sea salt

5 cups grated peeled zucchini (about 6 medium zucchini

½ cup ripe bananas

6 eggs, well beaten

½ cup butter, melted

½ cup honey

2 tsp vanilla flavoring or extract

Directions:

Preheat oven to 325°F.

Grease two 9-inch round cake pans and coat with flour. This can also be made in one 9-inch tube pan or a 9 x 5 x 3-inch loaf pan. Or, line two 12-cup muffin tins with paper liners and spray with oil spray.

Blend dry ingredients together so baking soda, baking powder, and xanthan gum are evenly distributed.

Mix all the wet ingredients together and then blend the wet into the dry—it Servings: a spongy mass, but don't worry.

Spoon batter into prepared cake pans.

Bake 45 to 60 minutes.

Cool on rack.

271. Tapioca White Cake

Preparation time: 15 minutes

Cooking time: 40 minutes

Servings: 12

Nutrition:

Carbohydrates – 24.9 g

Fat – 20.7 g

Protein – 3.9 g

Calories – 301

Ingredients:

4 eggs, separated and beaten

1 cup butter

2 tsp almond flavoring or extract

½ tsp cream of tartar

½ cup sugar

2 tsp vanilla flavoring or extract

1 cup tapioca flour

½ cup almond flour

½ tsp baking powder

½ tsp baking soda

1 tsp xanthan gum

Directions:

Preheat oven to 350°F.

Grease 9-inch tube pan and dust with tapioca flour.

Beat egg whites in a clean bowl until stiff, and gradually add cream of tartar.

Cream butter and sugar in a separate bowl.

Add vanilla, beaten egg yolks, and almond flavoring to the butter mixture.

Combine flours, baking powder, baking soda, and xanthan gum.

Add flour mixture to butter mixture and stir well.

Fold in egg whites.

Bake for 35-40 minutes or till done.

Invert pan on top of rack. Place a wet towel on pan bottom to help loosen the cake. Tap pan to loosen. Carefully nudge it out.

Cool cake upside down on a rack. Invert onto plate when cool.

272. Nut And Buckwheat Spice Cake

Preparation time: 15 minutes
Cooking time: 35 minutes
Servings: 12
Nutrition:
Carbohydrates – 56.4 g
Fat – 30.3 g
Protein – 6.5 g
Calories – 527
Ingredients:
1 cup buckwheat flour
½ cup bean flour
½ cup hazelnut flour
½ tsp xanthan gum
1 tsp baking powder
½ tsp baking soda
3 Tbsp ground cinnamon
2 Tbsp cumin
1 tsp sea salt
1 cup plain chopped nuts (pecans or walnuts
2 eggs
1 cup safflower oil or 1 cup unsalted butter, melted
1 cup honey
2 cups applesauce
Directions:
Preheat oven to 350°F.
Lightly grease two 8-inch round cake pans or one 11 x 7-inch cake pan.
Mix dry ingredients, except nuts, together.
Beat eggs until fluffy.
Combine the oil or butter and honey; add to the beaten eggs.
Add dry ingredients to wet ingredients (except applesauce). Beat just until smooth.
Mix in applesauce and nuts.
Pour cake mixture into baking pan or pans.
Bake for approximately 25 minutes (2 round pans for layer cakeor 35 minutes (single rectangular cake pan). Test with toothpick for doneness.

273. Teff Gingerbread

Preparation time: 15 minutes

Cooking time: 30 minutes

Servings: 16

Nutrition:

Carbohydrates – 15.7 g

Fat – 30.3 g

Protein – 2.2 g

Calories – 106

Ingredients:

1½ cups teff flour

½ cup quinoa flour

½ cup buckwheat flour

1 tsp baking powder

½ tsp baking soda

2 tsp xanthan gum

½ cup light brown sugar, packed, or granulated maple sugar

2 tsp cinnamon

2 tsp ground ginger or 3 tsp grated fresh ginger

½ tsp sea salt

1 tsp grated nutmeg

½ tsp allspice

½ tsp ground cloves

1 egg

4 Tbsp butter, melted

1 cup buttermilk

¼ cup unsulfured molasses (optional

Directions:

Preheat oven 425°F.

Grease a 9-inch square cake pan; dust with rice flour.

Blend dry ingredients in bowl.

Blend wet ingredients in another bowl.

Whisk wet ingredients into dry.

Bake for 30 minutes, or until toothpick inserted in center comes out dry.

274. Banana Cake

Preparation time: 15 minutes
Cooking time: 40 minutes
Servings: 16
Nutrition:
Carbohydrates – 35 g
Fat – 15.4 g
Protein – 8.4 g
Calories – 312
Ingredients:
1½ cups almond meal flour
1½ cups amaranth or sorghum flour
½ cup arrowroot
½ tsp sea salt
1 tsp baking powder
1 tsp baking soda
1 tsp xanthan gum
3 ripe bananas, mashed
2 Tbsp lemon juice
½ cup butter, melted
½ cup honey
3 eggs
2 tsp vanilla flavoring or extract
Directions:
Preheat oven to 350°F.
Grease 9-inch square pan; dust with rice flour.
Blend all dry ingredients in large mixing bowl.
Blend wet ingredients in a separate bowl using electric mixer.
Pour liquid ingredients over dry and stir gently.
Pour into baking dish.
Bake for 40 minutes; test with toothpick for doneness.

275. Cranberry Loaf Cake

Preparation time: 15 minutes

Cooking time: 40 minutes

Servings: 12

Nutrition:

Carbohydrates – 43 g

Fat – 14.6 g

Protein – 7.9 g

Calories – 336

Ingredients:

½ cup rice flour

1 cup almond meal flour

½ cup hazelnut flour

2 tsp nutmeg

1 tsp cumin

1½ tsp baking soda

1 cup GF dried cranberries

2 eggs, beaten till frothy

1 Tbsp oil

1 cup plain yogurt

½ cup GF rice syrup

½ cup orange juice

½ cup jam, marmalade, or conServings: (apricot, strawberry, pineapple, etc.

Directions:

Preheat oven to 350°F.

Grease one 8 x 4 x 3-inch loaf pan.

Mix dry ingredients (except fruittogether.

Mix wet ingredients (except jam, marmalade, or conservestogether.

Combine wet and dry ingredients. (Add a few more drops of juice or water if mixture is dry.

Fold dried fruit and preServings: into batter.

Bake in prepared loaf pan for 40 minutes or until top is golden.

276. Chocolate Dump-It Cake

Preparation time: 15 minutes

Cooking time: 25 minutes

Servings: 18

Nutrition:

Carbohydrates – 31.6 g

Fat – 4.5 g

Protein – 1.7 g

Calories – 174

Ingredients:

½ cup pure GF cocoa powder

½ cup boiling water

1 cup cornstarch

1½ cups potato starch

1 Tbsp plus 1½ tsp baking powder

1 tsp salt

1 cup sugar

1 can of cherry pie filling

2 eggs, beaten until frothy

½ cup canola oil

2 tsp vanilla flavoring or extract

2½ tsp guar gum or xanthan gum

1¼ cups milk, divided

Directions:

Preheat oven to 350°F.

Grease a 9 x 13- inch pan.

Combine cocoa powder and boiling water in a large bowl; mix well.

Add remaining ingredients, except for 1 cup milk. Mix well to remove all lumps from batter.

Add milk slowly. Mix just until combined. Add a little more milk if batter seems heavy.

Pour batter into prepared pan.

Bake for 22-25 minutes, until a toothpick inserted in the middle of the cake tests clean.

277. Carob Fudge Cake

Preparation time: 15 minutes

Cooking time: 30 minutes

Servings: 12

Nutrition:

Carbohydrates – 34.9 g

Fat – 8.6 g

Protein – 3.4 g

Calories – 231

Ingredients:

1 cup brown rice flour, sifted

½ cup amaranth flour, sifted

½ cup pure carob powder

1 tsp baking soda

½ tsp sea salt

½ cup plain nuts, chopped

½ cup warm water

½ cup oil

½ cup honey

1 Tbsp vinegar or lemon juice

1 tsp vanilla flavoring or extract

Directions:

Preheat oven to 350°F.

Grease 8-inch square baking pan; set aside.

 Combine dry ingredients, except nuts, in a bowl. Mix well, then sift into another bowl.

Combine wet ingredients in a small bowl. Mix together with fork or whisk.

Pour mixed wet ingredients over dry ingredients (all at once), then mix quickly.

Pour immediately into prepared baking pan. Scatter nuts on top of batter.

Bake 25 to 30 minutes. When done, cracks will (typicallyappear in top. The inside remains moist and fudgy.

278. Carrot Cake

Preparation time: 15 minutes

Cooking time: 50 minutes

Servings: 10

Nutrition:

Carbohydrates – 68.9 g

Fat – 27.9 g

Protein – 9.6 g

Calories – 565

Ingredients:

1½ cups teff flour

1 cup tapioca flour

½ cup fava bean flour

2 tsp xanthan gum

1 tsp baking soda

2 tsp cinnamon

2 tsp ground ginger

3 cups shredded carrots

1 cup plain pecans, chopped

½ cup butter, softened

1 cup brown sugar, packed, or 1 cup honey

4 eggs, at room temperature, beaten

1 cup plain yogurt

1 tsp vanilla flavoring or extract

1 cup crushed pineapple

Icing:

3 ounces GF cream cheese, softened

2 cups GF confectioners'sugar

2 Tbsp milk

1 tsp almond flavoring or extract

Directions:

Preheat oven to 350°F.

Grease a 9-inch springform or tube pan; dust with rice flour.

Combine flours, xanthan gum, baking powder, baking soda, cinnamon, and ginger together in bowl.

Cream together butter and sugar in a large bowl.

Whisk in eggs.

Add yogurt and vanilla, blend.

Add flour mixture to the egg mixture; stir just until blended.

Stir in carrots, pecans, and pineapple.

Pour batter into prepared pan.

Bake 45-50 minutes, until toothpick inserted in center comes out clean.

279. Hazelnut Applesauce Cake

Preparation time: 20 minutes
Cooking time: 40 minutes
Servings: 12
Nutrition:
Carbohydrates – 33.1 g
Fat – 19.1 g
Protein – 3.8 g
Calories – 319
Ingredients:
1½ cups hazelnut flour
1 cup currants or other GF dried fruit
½ cup plain pecans, chopped
½ cup bean flour
½ cup tapioca flour
½ tsp baking soda
½ tsp baking powder
½ tsp cream of tartar
½ tsp salt
1 tsp ground cloves
1 tsp xanthan gum
½ cup unsalted butter, melted
½ cup maple syrup
1 large egg, beaten
2 cups applesauce
Directions:
Preheat oven to 350°F.
Grease an 8-inch square cake pan and dust lightly with rice or quinoa flour.
Sprinkle some of the hazelnut flour over the fruit and nuts in separate bowl; toss until coated.
Blend remaining hazelnut flour with dry ingredients (except fruit and nuts).
Combine wet ingredients; mix well.
Mix wet ingredients into dry ingredients, blending well.
Fold nuts and fruit into the batter.
Spoon or pour batter into prepared cake pan.
Bake for 40 minutes or until toothpick comes out clean.

Chapter 6. Creative Combination Breads

280. Cream Cheese Stuffed Sweet Peppers

Serving: 12

Nutrition: 98.4 Cal; 7.4 g Fats; 5 g Protein; 0.9 g Net Carb; 2 g Fiber;

Ingredients

12 mini sweet peppers, halved, deseeded

8 ounces cream cheese, softened, full-fat

1/2 teaspoon paprika

1 teaspoon garlic powder

1/2 teaspoon ground black pepper

1/2 teaspoon salt

1/2 teaspoon red chili powder

1/2 teaspoon onion powder

2 tablespoons shredded cheddar cheese, full-fat

2 tablespoons shredded mozzarella cheese, full-fat

Directions

Switch on the oven, set it to 350 degrees F and let preheat.

Meanwhile, place all the ingredients in a bowl, except for mini peppers and stir until well mixed.

Spoon each mini pepper half with the cheese mixture until filled, then take a baking sheet, line it with parchment paper and place stuffed mini peppers on it.

Bake the mini peppers into the preheated oven for 20 minutes or until the top is lightly golden brown and peppers are soft.

Serve straight away.

281. Taco Stuffed Mini Peppers

Serving: 12

Nutrition: 319 Cal; 26 g Fats; 22 g Protein; 6 g Net Carb; 2 g Fiber;

Ingredients

1 pound ground beef, grass-fed

1 pound mini sweet peppers, halved, deseeded

10 ounces diced tomatoes with green chilies

2 tablespoons taco seasoning

8 ounces cream cheese, soften, full-fat

2 tablespoons hot sauce

1 cup grated cheddar cheese, full-fat, divided

2 tablespoons chopped cilantro

1 cup grated Monterey jack, full-fat, divided

Directions

Switch on the oven, set it to 350 degrees F and let preheat.

Meanwhile, take a skillet pan, place it over medium heat, and add beef and cook for 5 to 7 minutes or until thoroughly cooked.

Drain the fat from the pan, then add tomatoes, sprinkle with taco seasoning, add hot sauce, cream cheese and ½ cup each of cheddar and Monterey cheese, and continue cooking for 5 minutes at low heat until cheese has melted.

Remove pan from the heat, then stuff peppers with the beef mixture until filled and place them in a 9 by 13 inches baking dish.

Top peppers with remaining cheeses and bake the peppers for 10 minutes or until peppers are warm through.

Sprinkle cilantro over peppers and serve.

282. Chicken Stuffed Jalapeno Poppers

Serving: 4

Nutrition: 398.8 Cal; 34.6 g Fats; 18.5 g Protein; 0.6 g Net Carb; 1.6 g Fiber;

Ingredients

4 medium jalapeno peppers, halved and deseeded

2 strips of thick-cut bacon, pastured

1 ounce cooked chicken, pastured

¼ teaspoon ground black pepper

2 ounces cream cheese, full-fat

1 ounce shredded cheddar cheese, full-fat

Directions

Switch on the oven, set it to 375 degrees F and let preheat.

Meanwhile, place all the ingredients in a bowl, reserving peppers and bacon and stir until mixed.

Spoon the chicken mixture into peppers until filled, then cut bacon into four slices, lengthwise, and then wrap each pepper with a bacon strip, securing with a toothpick.

Take a baking tray, line it with aluminum foil, place stuffed and wrapped peppers on it and bake them for 15 to 20 minutes or until peppers are thoroughly cooked, and bacon is crispy.

Serve straight away.

283. Garlic Parmesan Wings

Serving: 6

Nutrition: 556 Cal; 42 g Fats; 36 g Protein; 4 g Net Carb; 0 g Fiber;

Ingredients

4 pounds chicken wings, pastured

2 tablespoons minced garlic

1 teaspoon ground black pepper

1 teaspoon salt

2 tablespoons baking powder

1 stick of butter, unsalted, melted

3/4 cup grated parmesan cheese, full-fat

Directions

Switch on the oven, set it to 250 degrees F and let preheat.

Meanwhile, place half of the chicken wings in a plastic bag, add half of salt and baking powder, then seal the bag and toss the chicken wings until well coated.

Lay the coated chicken wings on a rack placed in a baking pan, then coat remaining chicken wings in the same manner and place them on the rack as well.

Bake the chicken wings in the center rack of the preheated oven for 30 minutes, then flip the wings and continue baking the chicken wings for 40 minutes at 425 degrees F.

Meanwhile, whisk together remaining ingredients in a large bowl until combined and set aside until required.

When the chicken wings have baked, transfer them to the bowl containing cheese mixture by using a tong and toss until evenly coated.

Serve straight away.

284. Bacon-Wrapped Parmesan Chicken

Serving: 6

Nutrition: 239 Cal; 14.2 g Fats; 52.7 g Protein; 0.83 g Net Carb; 0 g Fiber;

Ingredients

bacon slices, pastured, as needed per chicken strip

1 pound chicken breast, pastured, cut into strips

½ teaspoon ground black pepper

1 teaspoon salt

2 tablespoons avocado oil

1 cup grated parmesan cheese, full-fat

2 eggs, pastured

Directions

Crack the eggs in a bowl and then whisk until blended, set aside until required.

Place cheese in another bowl, add salt and black pepper and stir until combined, set aside until required.

Take a large skillet, place it over medium heat, grease with avocado oil and let heat.

Meanwhile, dip a chicken strip into the egg, then coat with parmesan cheese mixture and wrap with a bacon slice, prepare the remaining chicken strips in the same manner.

Add chicken strips into the heated pan in single layer and cook for 4 minutes per side or until thoroughly cooked.

Serve straight away.

285. Sausage And Cheese Dip

Serving:

Nutrition: 2240 Cal; 189 g Fats; 124 g Protein; 4 g Net Carb; 0 g Fiber;

Ingredients

10 ounces diced tomatoes

1 pound hot sausage, pastured

4.5 ounces diced green chilies

1/2 teaspoon red pepper flakes

1 teaspoon garlic powder

1/4 teaspoon cumin

8 ounces cream cheese, full-fat

1 cup grated cheddar cheese, full-fat

1 cup grated Monterrey jack cheese, full-fat

Directions

Switch on the oven, set it to 350 degrees F and let preheat.

Meanwhile, take a skillet pan, place it over medium heat, add sausage and cook for 5 to 7 minutes or until cooked.

Drain the fats from the pan, add cream cheese, stir until combined, then add remaining ingredients and stir until well combined.

Turn heat to medium-low level and cook the dip for 5 to 7 minutes or until cheese has melted and dip is smooth.

Turn heat to the low level, cover the pan with lid and then simmer the dip for 5 minutes.

Serve the dip with sliced veggies.

286. Creamy Spinach Dip

Serving: 6

Nutrition: 312 Cal; 34 g Fats; 1 g Protein; 2 g Net Carb; 1 g Fiber;

Ingredients

2 ounces frozen spinach

2 tablespoons avocado oil

2 tablespoons dried parsley

1 teaspoon onion powder

¼ teaspoon ground black pepper

½ teaspoon salt

1 tablespoon dried dill

2 tsp lemon juice

1 cup mayonnaise, full-fat

¼ cup sour cream, full-fat

Directions

Thaw the spinach, then squeeze moisture from it as much as possible and then place in a bowl.

Add remaining ingredients, then stir until well mixed and let the dip sit at room temperature for 10 minutes.

Serve straight away.

287. Dill Pickle Dip

Serving: 10

Nutrition: 87 Cal; 9 g Fats; 1 g Protein; 2 g Net Carb; 0 g Fiber;

Ingredients

8 ounces cream cheese, softened, full-fat

1 1/2 cups chopped dill pickles

1/2 teaspoon onion powder

1/2 teaspoon garlic powder

½ teaspoon ground black pepper

½ teaspoon salt

1/4 cup chopped dill

1/2 cup sour cream, full-fat

3 tablespoons pickle juice

Directions

Place pickles in a food processor, pulse until chopped and then tip the mixture in a bowl.

Add remaining ingredients and then stir until well combined.

Serve straight away.

288. Zucchini Fries With Avocado Dip

Serving: 3

Nutrition: 376 Cal; 32 g Fats; 12 g Protein; 7 g Net Carb; 3 g Fiber;

Ingredients

For The Zucchini Fries:

2 large zucchinis

½ cup shredded coconut, unsweetened

½ cup almond flour

1 teaspoon garlic powder

1 teaspoon smoked paprika

1 teaspoon ground cumin

¾ teaspoon salt

2 eggs, pastured

For The Sauce:

1 medium avocado, pitted

½ tablespoon minced garlic

1 teaspoon hot sauce, sugar-free

¼ teaspoon salt

1 tablespoon lime juice

2 tablespoons yogurt, high-fat

Water as needed to thin

Directions

Switch on the oven, set it to 450 degrees F and let preheat.

Meanwhile, cut each zucchini in half, lengthwise, then crosswise and into small wedges, set aside until required.

Place shredded coconut in a food processor, pulse until coconut resembles fine sand, then tip it in a bowl, add flour, garlic, salt, cumin and paprika and stir until mixed.

Crack the eggs in another bowl and then whisk until blended.

Working on one zucchini wedge at a time, first dip it into the egg, then coat with almond flour mixture and then place onto prepared baking sheet.

Coat the remaining zucchini wedges in the same manner and then place them onto the baking sheets in a single layer.

Bake zucchini wedges for 15 minutes or until nicely golden brown.

Meanwhile, prepare the dip and for this, place all the ingredients for the dip in a food processor and blend until smooth, slowly blending in water until dip reaches to desired consistency.

Serve zucchini wedges with prepared dip.

289. Pizza Bites

Serving: 30

Nutrition: 82 Cal; 7 g Fats; 3.9 g Protein; 0.8 g Net Carb; 0.5 g Fiber;

Ingredients

1/3 cup coconut flour

1 pound Italian sausage, pastured, cooked and drained

1 teaspoon Italian seasoning

1/2 teaspoon baking powder

1 teaspoon minced garlic

3 eggs, pastured, beaten

4 ounces cream cheese, full-fat, softened

1 1/4 cup shredded mozzarella cheese, full-fat

Directions

Switch on the oven, set it to 350 degrees F and let preheat.

Meanwhile, place sausage and cream cheese in a large bowl, stir until combined, then add remaining ingredients and stir until well mixed.

Place the bowl in the refrigerator and let the mixture chill for 10 minutes.

Then take a baking sheet, grease it with oil, drop sausage mixture on it by using a small cookie scoop and bake for 20 minutes or until nicely golden brown.

Serve straight away.

290. Buffalo Chicken Dip

Serving: 4

Nutrition: 415.5 Cal; 28.6 g Fats; 35.3 g Protein; 3.7 g Net Carb; 2.3 g Fiber;

Ingredients

2 cups cooked chicken, pastured, shredded

8 ounces cream cheese, full-fat, softened

1/2 cup sour cream, full-fat

1/2 cup Frank's red hot sauce, full-fat

1 ½ tablespoon snipped chives

Directions

Switch on the oven, set it to 350 degrees F and let preheat.

Meanwhile, place all the ingredients in a bowl, except for chives, and stir until well mixed.

Take an 8 by 8 inches casserole dish, place the chicken dip mixture in it and bake for 20 to 25 minutes or until dip bubbles.

Then switch on the broiler and continue cooking for 5 minutes or until the top is nicely brown and crispy.

Sprinkle chives on the dip and then serve the dip straight away with celery.

291. Buffalo Deviled Eggs

Serving: 6

Nutrition: 167 Cal; 14 g Fats; 8.6 g Protein; 1.2 g Net Carb; 1.3 g Fiber;

Ingredients

1 celery stalk

3 tablespoons mayonnaise, full-fat

1/3 cup crumbled blue cheese, full-fat

2 tablespoons buffalo sauce, full-fat

6 eggs, pastured, boiled

1 tablespoon chopped chives

Directions

Peel the boiled eggs, then cut into half lengthwise, transfer their yolks into a bowl and add mayonnaise and buffalo sauce and stir until well combined.

Transfer the yolks mixture in a piping bag and then stuff each egg white with it until filled.

Top each deviled egg with sauce, cheese, celery, and chives and then serve.

292. Pickled Deviled Eggs

Serving: 12

Nutrition: 55 Cal; 4 g Fats; 2.5 g Protein; 2 g Net Carb; 0 g Fiber;

Ingredients

1/4 cup chopped pickle

2 teaspoons chopped dill

¼ teaspoon paprika

¼ teaspoon ground black pepper

¼ teaspoon salt

1 tablespoon pickle juice

6 eggs, pastured, boiled

3 tablespoons mayonnaise, full-fat

1 teaspoon Dijon mustard

Directions

Peel the boiled eggs, then cut into half lengthwise and transfer their yolks into a bowl.

Add remaining ingredients, except for paprika, then stir until well combined and transfer the yolks mixture in a piping bag.

Stuff each egg white with the yolk mixture until filled, then garnish with paprika and serve.

293. Lettuce Wraps

Serving: 6

Nutrition: 136 Cal; 10 g Fats; 10 g Protein; 1 g Net Carb; 0.5 g Fiber;

Ingredients

1/3 cup bacon bits, pastured

8 ounces cooked rotisserie chicken, cut into cubed

2 heads of romaine lettuce, leaves separated

2 tomatoes, diced

3 tablespoons mayonnaise, full-fat

3 tablespoons ranch dressing, low-carb

1/3 cup of shredded cheddar cheese, full-fat

Directions

Place chicken cubes in a bowl, add bacon, cheese and mayonnaise and toss until well combined.

Then take out the leaves from the heads of lettuce, about 12 twelve, then make a holder for chicken mixture by using a pair of leaves and evenly divide with chicken mixture.

Top with tomatoes, then drizzle with ranch dressing and serve.

294. Chili Lime Beef Jerky

Serving: 8

Nutrition: 137 Cal; 6 g Fats; 17 g Protein; 0.9 g Net Carb; 0.4 g Fiber;

Ingredients

1 pound flank steak, pastured

1 tablespoon garlic powder

1 tablespoon salt

1 tablespoon red chili powder

1/2 teaspoon ground black pepper

Directions

Switch on the oven, set it to 225 degrees F and let preheat.

Meanwhile, cut the beef into 2-inch wide strips, about 1/8-inch thick and then pound each beef strip with a meat mallet until evenly thick.

Then place the beef strips in a large bowl, add remaining ingredients and toss until well coated.

Take two baking sheets, line them with parchment paper, and then place coated beef strips in a single layer and bake for 3 hours until beef strips are dry and nicely browned, rotating the baking sheets halfway through.

When done, transfer beef strips onto a cooling rack and let cool for 1 hour or until dry.

Serve straight away.

295. Stuffed Mushrooms

Serving: 4

Nutrition: 164 Cal; 12 g Fats; 9 g Protein; 2 g Net Carb; 2 g Fiber;

Ingredients

1 pound mushrooms, about 20

1 ½ tablespoon minced garlic

1 tablespoon fresh chopped parsley

1/4 teaspoon ground black pepper

1/2 teaspoon salt

1 tablespoon butter, unsalted, softened

3/4 cup shredded cheddar cheese

2 tablespoons cream cheese, full-fat, softened

Directions

Switch on the oven, set it to 390 degrees F and let preheat.

Meanwhile, remove the stalk from each pepper, then peel the skins and set them aside until required.

Place cream cheese in a bowl, add garlic, butter, and parsley and stir until well mixed.

Add remaining ingredients, stir until combined and then stuff each mushroom with the cheese mixture until filled.

Place stuffed mushrooms on a cookie sheet lined with parchment sheet and then bake them for 15 minutes or until mushrooms are thoroughly cooked, and cheese are nicely golden brown.

Serve straight away.

296. Pretzels

Serving: 4

Nutrition: 363.25 Cal; 32.4 g Fats; 17.35 g Protein; 3.2 g Net Carb; 2.2 g Fiber;

Ingredients

For The Pretzel Dough:

3/4 cup almond flour

1 1/2 tsp garlic powder

1 tsp Italian seasoning

1 egg, pastured, beaten

1 1/2 cup shredded mozzarella cheese, full-fat

2 tablespoons cream cheese, full-fat

For The Garlic Parmesan Topping:

1 1/2 teaspoons garlic powder

1 teaspoon Italian seasoning

4 tablespoons grated parmesan cheese, full-fat

3 tablespoons butter, unsalted, melted

Directions

Switch on the oven, set it to 350 degrees F and let preheat.

Meanwhile, place cream cheese and mozzarella cheese in a heatproof bowl and microwave for 1 minute or until cheese has melted, stirring halfway through.

Then let the cheese cool for 5 minutes, add flour along with Italian seasoning and garlic powder and beat in eggs until incorporated.

Divide the dough evenly between four sections, then shape each dough section into pretzel and place on a baking sheet lined with parchment paper.

Brush each pretzel dough generously with butter, sprinkle with garlic powder, Italian seasoning, and parmesan cheese and bake the pretzels for 15 minutes or until nicely golden brown.

Serve straight away.

297. Popcorn Chicken Bites

Serving: 4

Nutrition: 253.7 Cal; 18.9 g Fats; 16.9 g Protein; 2.2 g Net Carb; 3.4 g Fiber;

Ingredients

1 1/2 cup almond flour

1 pound chicken breast, pastured, cut into cubes

1 teaspoon onion powder

1/2 teaspoon ground black pepper

1/2 teaspoon salt

1 teaspoon garlic powder

1 teaspoon red chili powder

1 teaspoon cayenne pepper

1 teaspoon paprika

1 1/2 teaspoon red pepper flakes

1 egg, pastured

Directions

Switch on the oven, set it to 400 degrees F and let preheat.

Meanwhile, cut the chicken into large bite-size pieces and set aside until required.

Crack the egg in a bowl and then whisk until blended, set aside until required.

Place almond flour in another bowl, add remaining ingredients and then stir until well combined.

Dip some chicken cubes into the egg, then transfer them into bowl containing almond flour mixture, cover the bowl with lid and shake well until the chicken cubes are well coated.

Place the coated chicken cubes on a baking sheet lined with foil, then coat remaining chicken cubes in batches in the same manner and place them onto the baking sheet.

Bake the chicken cubes for 20 minutes or until crispy and thoroughly cooked, then switch on the broiler and continue cooking for 2 minutes.

Serve straight away.

298. Mug Biscuit

Serving: 1

Nutrition: 330 Cal; 26 g Fats; 12 g Protein; 7 g Net Carb; 5 g Fiber;

Ingredients

1 tablespoon coconut flour

1 teaspoon swerve sweetener

¼ teaspoon baking powder

1/8 teaspoon salt

3 tablespoons almond flour

2 teaspoons avocado oil

1 egg, pastured

Directions

Take a heatproof mug, add flours, sweetener, baking powder, and salt and stir until well combined.

Add oil and egg, whisk until incorporated and microwave for 1 minute at high heat setting or until biscuit is cooked and puffed.

Take out the biscuit, cut in half from the middle, then smear it with butter and serve.

299. Coconut Flour Biscuits

Serving: 7

Nutrition: 133 Cal; 10.1 g Fats; 5.4 g Protein; 1.4 g Net Carb; 3 g Fiber;

Ingredients

½ cup coconut flour

¼ teaspoon baking soda

4 eggs, pastured

¼ cup melted butter, unsalted

Directions

Switch on the oven, set it to 350 degrees F and let preheat.

Meanwhile, place the flour in a bowl, add baking soda and stir until well mixed.

Stir in butter until combined and whisk in the egg until incorporated.

Take a baking sheet, grease it with avocado oil, then scoop the mixture on it, about 3 tablespoons per biscuit, and bake for 20 minutes or until biscuits are nicely golden brown.

Serve straight away.

300. Simple Keto Biscuits

Serving: 10

Nutrition: 116 Cal; 9.8 g Fats; 5 g Protein; 1 g Net Carb; 0 g Fiber;

Ingredients

6 ounces almond butter, unsweetened, softened

1 egg, pastured

2.4 ounces erythritol sweetener

½ teaspoon liquid stevia

Directions

Switch on the oven, set it to 350 degrees F and let preheat.

Meanwhile, place the butter in a bowl, beat until creamy, and then beat in egg and sweeteners until incorporated.

Take a baking sheet, grease it with avocado oil, then divide the prepared dough into ten sections, and roll each section into a ball.

Place the dough balls onto the baking sheet, flatten them slightly and bake for 12 minutes or until biscuits are nicely golden brown.

When the biscuits have baked, let them cool completely on a wire rack and then serve.

301. Cheesy Biscuits

Serving: 9

Nutrition: 329 Cal; 27.1 g Fats; 16.7 g Protein; 4.1 g Net Carb; 2.9 g Fiber;

Ingredients

2 cups almond flour

1 tablespoon baking powder

4 eggs, pastured

2 1/2 cups grated cheddar cheese, full-fat

1/4 cup half-and-half, grass-fed, full-fat

Directions

Switch on the oven, set it to 350 degrees F and let preheat.

Meanwhile, place flour in a bowl, stir in baking powder, add cheese and stir until well mixed.

Make a well in the center of the bowl, add half-and-half and eggs and stir well by using a flour until sticky batter comes together.

Take a baking sheet, grease it with avocado oil, then scoop the batter on it, about nine portions and bake for 20 minutes or until nicely golden brown.

Let biscuits cool for 30 minutes and then serve.

302. Almond Flour Biscuits

Serving: 12

Nutrition: 164 Cal; 15 g Fats; 5 g Protein; 2 g Net Carb; 2 g Fiber;

Ingredients

2 cups almond flour

1/2 teaspoon sea salt

2 teaspoons baking powder

1/3 cup butter, unsalted

2 eggs, pastured, beaten

Directions

Switch on the oven, set it to 350 degrees F and let preheat.

Meanwhile, place flour in a bowl, add salt and baking powder, stir until well combined, then add butter and eggs and whisk well until incorporated.

Take a baking sheet, grease it with avocado oil, then scoop the batter on it, about twelve portions, shape them into round biscuits and bake for 15 minutes or until nicely golden brown.

Let biscuits cool in the baking sheet and then serve.

303. Sour Cream Biscuits

Serving: 4

Nutrition: 251.2 Cal; 22 g Fats; 7.5 g Protein; 3.4 g Net Carb; 2.3 g Fiber;

Ingredients

1 cup almond flour

1/2 teaspoon xanthan gum

1/4 teaspoon sea salt

1 teaspoon baking powder

1 tablespoon ground flax seeds

2 tablespoons butter, unsalted, cut into chunks

1 egg white, pastured

2 tablespoons sour cream, grass-fed, full-fat

Directions

Switch on the oven, set it to 400 degrees F and let preheat.

Meanwhile, place flour in a food processor, add flaxseed, salt, baking powder, and xanthan gum and stir until mixed.

Add butter, pulse more or until mixture resembles crumbs and then tip the mixture in a bowl.

Place egg white in a bowl, add sour cream, whisk until combined, add into flour mixture and stir well until incorporated and the dough comes together.

Place a piece of parchment sheet on a working place, place the dough on it, then shape it into a ½-inch dish, then cut into desired shape biscuits and place on a baking sheet lined with parchment sheet, 2-inches apart.

Bake the biscuits for 10 to 12 minutes or until nicely golden brown and then let them cool.

Serve straight away.

304. Mozzarella Bagels

Serving: 6

Nutrition: 203 Cal; 16.8 g Fats; 11 g Protein; 2.4 g Net Carb; 1.6 g Fiber;

Ingredients

3/4 cup almond meal

¼ teaspoon salt

1 teaspoon baking powder

1 3/4 cup grated mozzarella cheese, full-fat

1 egg, pastured

2 tablespoons cream cheese, grass-fed, full-fat

Directions

Switch on the oven, set it to 350 degrees F and let preheat.

Meanwhile, place cream cheese in a heatproof bowl, add mozzarella cheese and microwave for 30 seconds or until cheese has melted, stirring halfway through.

Then add egg into melted cheeses along with salt and baking powder and stir well until incorporated and the dough comes together.

Divide the dough into six sections, roll each section into a log, then form a bagel shape by folding the ends of each log in a circle and squeezing the ends together.

Place bagels onto a baking sheet lined with parchment paper and then bake for 15 minutes or until golden brown.

Serve straight away.

305. Almond Flour Bagels

Serving: 8

Nutrition: 271 Cal; 22 g Fats; 13 g Protein; 2 g Net Carb; 2 g Fiber;

Ingredients

1 3/4 cups almond flour

1/4 teaspoon salt

2 teaspoons baking powder

2 ounces cream cheese, grass-fed, full-fat

2 eggs, pastured, beaten

2 cups shredded mozzarella cheese, full-fat

1 egg yolk, pastured

3 tablespoons sesame seeds

Directions

Switch on the oven, set it to 415 degrees F and let preheat.

Meanwhile, place flour in a bowl, add salt and baking powder and stir until mixed, set aside until required.

Place the egg yolk in a bowl, add water, whisk well until blended and set aside until required.

Place cream cheese in a heatproof bowl, add mozzarella cheese and microwave for 30 seconds or until cheese has melted, stirring halfway through.

Add melted cheese into the flour, stir until combined, then beat in eggs and knead the mixture until a smooth dough comes together.

Divide the dough into eight sections, roll each section in a log, shape it into a bagel and place on a baking sheet, lined with parchment sheet.

Brush each bagel with an egg wash, sprinkle with sesame seeds and bake for 15 minutes or until golden.

Let the bagels cool on a wire rack and then serve.

306. Cinnamon Bagel Bites

Serving: 16

Nutrition: 94.8 Cal; 7 g Fats; 5.4 g Protein; 1.9 g Net Carb; 1 g Fiber;

Ingredients

1 cup almond flour

2 teaspoon baking powder

3 tablespoons swerve sweetener

3 tablespoons coconut flour

1 teaspoon vanilla extract, unsweetened

1 1/2 cup shredded mozzarella cheese, full-fat

1 egg, pastured, beaten

2 ounces cream cheese, grass-fed, full-fat

For the Coating:

1 tablespoon swerve sweetener

2 teaspoons cinnamon

1 tablespoon melted butter, unsalted

Directions

Switch on the oven, set it to 400 degrees F and let preheat.

Meanwhile, place cream cheese in a heatproof bowl, add mozzarella cheese and microwave for 1 minute or until cheese has melted, stirring halfway through.

Meanwhile, place flours in a bowl, add baking powder and sweetener and stir until well mixed.

Then stir in cheese until incorporated, knead the mixture, then beat in vanilla and egg using an immersion blender until the dough comes together.

Refrigerate the dough for 10 minutes, then divide into sixteen sections, and roll each section into a ball.

Prepare the coating and for this, place sweetener and cinnamon in a shallow dish and stir until combined.

Brush each dough ball with butter generously, then roll it in the cinnamon mixture until well coated, place onto a baking sheet greased with avocado oil and bake for 10 minutes or until nicely golden brown.

Serve straight away.

307. Creamy Chocolate Muffins

Preparation time: 10 minutes
Cooking time: 11 minutes

Servings: 12
Ingredients:
1 cup creamy almond butter
2/3 cup erythritol
2 tbsp unsweetened cocoa powder
2 tbsp peanut butter powder
2 large eggs
1 tbsp salted butter, melted
2 tbsp water
1 1/2 tsp pure vanilla extract
1 tsp baking soda
1/4 cup sugar-free dark chocolate baking chips
How to prepare:
Start by preheating the oven to 350 degrees F.
Place a silicone muffin tray on a baking sheet.
Place almond butter in a mixing bowl and whisk in all other ingredients except chocolate chips.
Mix well until combined then fold in chocolate chips.
Divide the dough into 12 muffin cups.
Bake the muffins for 11 minutes, approximately.
Serve.
Nutrition:
Calories 139
Total Fat 4.6 g
Saturated Fat 0.5 g
Cholesterol 1.2 mg
Sodium 83 mg
Total Carbs 7.5 g
Sugar 6.3 g
Fiber 0.6 g
Protein 3.8 g

308. Pumpkin Spice Muffins

Preparation time: 10 minutes
Cooking time: 20 minutes

Servings: 6
Ingredients:
2/3 cup almond flour
3 tbsp coconut flour
1 tbsp psyllium husk
1 tsp pumpkin pie spice
1/2 tsp xanthan gum
1/4 tsp kosher salt
1/2 tsp baking powder
1/2 tsp baking soda
2 eggs, separated
1/3 cup golden erythritol
1 tsp vanilla extract
1 tsp apple cider vinegar
1/4 cup unsalted butter, melted
1/4 cup espresso, cooled
How to prepare:
Start by preheating the oven to 350 degrees F.
Whisk all the dry ingredients in a bowl and beat the wet ingredients
separately until fluffy.
Mix the two mixtures together then divide the batter into the muffin cups.
Bake them for 20 minutes or until golden brown.
Allow them to cool then serve.
Nutrition:
Calories 261
Total Fat 7.1 g
Saturated Fat 13.4 g
Cholesterol 0.3 mg
Sodium 10 mg
Total Carbs 6.1 g
Sugar 2.1 g
Fiber 3.9 g
Protein 1.8 g

309. Chocolate Zucchini Muffins

Preparation time: 10 minutes
Cooking time: 18 minutes

Servings: 8
Ingredients:
Dry Ingredients
3/4 cup Bob's Red Mill coconut flour
1/2 cup Swerve, granulated
1/4 cup cocoa powder
1 tbsp baking powder
1/2 tsp instant coffee granules
1/4 tsp xanthan gum
1/4 tsp salt
5 oz zucchini (about 1 small-medium zucchini
4 oz butter
1 oz unsweetened baking chocolate
Wet ingredients
6 large eggs
1/2 tsp vanilla
1/2 tsp stevia
1/4 cup chocolate chips
How to prepare:
Start by preheating the oven to 350 degrees F and set its rack in the middle.
Grease 12 muffin cups with cooking oil and set it aside.
Place the grated zucchini in a colander and sprinkle salt on top.
Let it sit for 15 minutes then squeeze out all the excess liquid and set aside.
Add all dry ingredients except zucchini, chocolate, and butter to a mixing bowl and set it aside.
Melt butter with chocolate in a microwave by heating it for 30 seconds.
Beat the wet ingredients in a bowl.
Stir in chocolate melt and dry mixture.
Mix until well incorporated then fold in zucchini.
Divide the prepared batter into the muffin cups and bake for 18 minutes.

Serve.

Nutrition:

Calories 151

Total Fat 14.7 g

Saturated Fat 1.5 g

Cholesterol 13 mg

Sodium 53 mg

Total Carbs 1.5 g

Sugar 0.3 g

Fiber 0.1 g

Protein 0.8 g

310. Cheesy Herb Muffins

Preparation time: 10 minutes
Cooking time: 22 minutes

Servings: 12
Ingredients:
6 tbsp butter
1 tsp granulated erythritol sweetener
1 cup superfine blanched almond flour
3 tbsp coconut flour
3/4 tsp kosher salt
1/4 tsp garlic powder
2 tsp baking powder
¼ tsp xanthan gum
2 eggs
1/2 tsp fresh thyme leaves
1/3 cup unsweetened almond milk
1/2 cup cheddar cheese, shredded
How to prepare:
Start by preheating the oven to 375 degrees F. Grease a muffin tray with cooking spray.
Melt butter in a bowl by heating in a microwave for 30 seconds.
Stir in almond flour, sweetener, garlic powder, eggs, and all other remaining ingredients.
Divide the prepared batter into the muffin cups and bake for 22 minutes, approximately.
Serve.
Nutrition:
Calories 195
Total Fat 14.3 g
Saturated Fat 10.5 g
Cholesterol 175 mg
Sodium 125 mg
Total Carbs 4.5 g
Sugar 0.5 g
Fiber 0.3 g
Protein 3.2 g

311. Lemon Poppy Seed Muffins

Preparation time: 10 minutes
Cooking time: 20 minutes

Servings: 6
Ingredients:
¾ cup almond flour
¼ cup golden flaxseed meal
1/3 cup erythritol
1 tsp baking powder
2 tbsp poppy seeds
¼ cup salted butter, melted
¼ cup heavy cream
3 large eggs
2 lemons, zested
3 tbsp lemon juice
1 tsp vanilla extract
25 drops liquid Stevia
How to prepare:
Start by preheating the oven to 350 degrees F.
Add poppy seeds, erythritol, flaxseed meal, and almond flour in a bowl.
Stir in eggs, cream, and melted butter then beat the mixture together.
Add Stevia, baking powder, lemon zest, lemon juice, and vanilla extract.
Divide the batter evenly into a muffin tray.
Bake them for 20 minutes or until golden brown on the top.
Serve.
Nutrition:
Calories 252
Total Fat 17.3 g
Saturated Fat 11.5 g
Cholesterol 141 mg
Sodium 153 mg
Total Carbs 7.2 g
Sugar 0.3 g
Fiber 1.4 g
Protein 5.2 g

312. Sesame Buns

Preparation time: 10 minutes
Cooking time: 25 minutes

Servings: 4
Ingredients:
3 egg whites, room temperature
1 egg, room temperature
1/4 cup boiling hot water
1/4 cup almond flour
1/4 cup coconut flour
1 tbsp psyllium husk powder
1 tsp baking powder
Sesame seeds, for sprinkling (optional
How to prepare:
Start by preheating the oven to 356 degrees F.
Throw all the dry ingredients into a food processor and mix together.
Add rest of the ingredients then blend well until smooth.
Divide the dough into 4 equal parts to make the buns.
Arrange them on a baking sheet lined with parchment sheet.
Sprinkle sesame seeds on top then bake them for 25 minutes until golden.
Serve.
Nutrition:
Calories 193
Total Fat 10 g
Saturated Fat 13.2 g
Cholesterol 120 mg
Sodium 8 mg
Total Carbs 2.5 g
Sugar 1 g
Fiber 0.7 g
Protein 2.2 g

313. Chocolate Swirl Buns

Preparation time: 10 minutes
Cooking time: 20 minutes

Servings: 6
Ingredients:
3/4 cup almond flour
1.5 cups mozzarella cheese, melted
1 scoop whey isolate
2 tsp baking powder
1/2 cup + 3 tbsp sugar substitute
1 medium egg
1 tbsp vanilla
1/4 cup melted butter
2 tbsp cocoa powder
1 handful of sugar-free chocolate chips
How to prepare:
Whisk almond flour with sweetener and baking powder in a mixing bowl.
Stir in vanilla, melted mozzarella, and the egg.
Mix well until it forms a smooth dough then spread the dough out in between two parchment sheets.
Brush the sheet with melt butter and drizzle the sweetener on top.
Add chocolate chips and cocoa powder over the sheet.
Roll the dough into a log and cut it into slices.
Arrange the slices on a baking sheet and bake them for 20 minutes approximately at 350 degrees F.
Serve.
Nutrition:
Calories 76
Total Fat 7.2 g
Saturated Fat 6.4 g
Cholesterol 134 mg
Sodium 8 mg
Total Carbs 2g
Sugar 1 g
Fiber 0.7 g
Protein 2.2 g

314. Hot Dog Buns

Preparation time: 10 minutes

Cooking time: 2 minutes

Servings: 11

Ingredients:

3/4 cup almond flour

3 large eggs

1 1/2 tsp baking powder

4 tbsp oil

How to prepare:

Throw all the ingredients into a casserole dish and mix well.

Place it in the microwave and cook for 2 minutes.

Slice the bread and serve with sausage.

Nutrition:

Calories 136

Total Fat 10.7 g

Saturated Fat 0.5 g

Cholesterol 4 mg

Sodium 45 mg

Total Carbs 1.2 g

Sugar 1.4 g

Fiber 0.2 g

Protein 0.9

315. Hamburger Bun

Preparation time: 10 minutes
Cooking time: 2 minutes

Servings: 1
Ingredients:
1 large egg
1 tbsp almond flour
1 tbsp psyllium husk powder
¼ tsp baking powder
¼ tsp cream of tartar
1 tbsp chicken broth
1 tbsp melted butter
How to prepare:
Crack an egg in a wide mug.

Melt butter in a separate bowl by heating for 15 seconds in the microwave.

Pour this butter over the egg then beat well.

Whisk well then add almond flour, baking powder, psyllium husk powder, chicken broth, and cream of tartar.

Beat well, and cook for 60 seconds in the microwave.

Remove, slice, and serve.

Nutrition:
Calories 200
Total Fat 11.1 g
Saturated Fat 9.5 g
Cholesterol 124.2 mg
Sodium 46 mg
Total Carbs 1.1 g
Sugar 1.3 g
Fiber 0.4 g
Protein 0.4 g

316. Spinach Buns

Preparation time: 10 minutes

Cooking time: 25 minutes

Servings: 4

Ingredients:

5 large eggs

1 cup packed spinach

¼ cup of coconut oil

1/3 cup coconut flour

½ tsp salt

1/2 tsp garlic powder

1/2 tsp baking soda

How to prepare:

Start by preheating the oven to 400 degrees F and layer a baking sheet with parchment paper.

Beat eggs with spinach and fat in a blender until smooth.

Stir in 1/3 cup coconut flour, baking soda, salt, and garlic powder.

Mix well to form a dough.

Divide the dough into 4 parts and roll them into balls.

Place them on the baking sheet then bake for 25 minutes until fluffy and golden brown.

Serve.

Nutrition:

Calories 139

Total Fat 4.6 g

Saturated Fat 0.5 g

Cholesterol 1.2 mg

Sodium 83 mg

Total Carbs 7.5 g

Sugar 6.3 g

Fiber 0.6 g

Protein 3.8 g

317. Pecan Fat Bombs

Preparation time: 10 minutes

Cooking time: 5 minutes

Cooking Time: 2 hours

Servings: 9

Ingredients:

4 oz unsalted butter

2 oz pecan butter

1 scoop vanilla collagen powder

2 tbsp sugar-free maple syrup

9 pecan nuts

How to prepare:

Throw all the ingredients except pecans into a saucepan.

Stir cook them on low heat for 5 minutes then remove from the heat.

Allow the mixture to cool for 5 minutes then divide the mixture into silicone molds.

Place a pecan at the center of each silicone mold.

Refrigerate the fat bombs for 2 hours.

Serve.

Nutrition:

Calories 113

Total Fat 9 g

Saturated Fat 0.2 g

Cholesterol 1.7 mg

Sodium 134 mg

Total Carbs 6.5 g

Sugar 1.8 g

Fiber 0.7 g

Protein 7.5 g

318. Chocolate Fat Bomb

Preparation time: 10 minutes
Cooking time: 3 hours

Servings: 12
Ingredients:
8 oz of cream cheese, softened
2 oz Natvia icing mix
1 tsp of vanilla essence
7 oz of heavy cream
5 oz of sugar-free chocolate
How to prepare:
Melt chocolate in a bowl by heating in a microwave for 1 minute.
Add cream cheese, vanilla essence, cream, and Natvia icing mix.
Beat well and transfer the mixture to a piping bag.
Pipe it evenly into 24 paper cupcakes and refrigerate for 3 hours.
Serve.
Nutrition:
Calories 117
Total Fat 21.2 g
Saturated Fat 10.4 g
Cholesterol 19.7 mg
Sodium 104 mg
Total Carbs 7.3 g
Sugar 3.4 g
Fiber 2 g
Protein 8.1 g

319. Keto Strawberry Fudge

Preparation time: 10 minutes

Cooking time: 1 hour

Total time: 1 hour 10 minutes

Servings: 6

Ingredients:

Vanilla Layer

8 oz cream cheese

8 oz butter

1 tbsp vanilla extract

2 tbsp erythritol

Strawberry Fudge Layer

8 oz cream cheese

8 oz butter

1 oz protein powder

How to prepare:

Start by lining a baking tray with parchment paper.

Mix cream cheese with vanilla extract, softened butter, and erythritol in a bowl.

Blend well on low speed then divide it into silicone molds.

Blend all the ingredients for the strawberry layer in a blender on low speed.

Divide this mixture into the silicone molds over the vanilla layer.

Refrigerate for 1 hour then serve.

Nutrition:

Calories 213

Total Fat 19 g

Saturated Fat 15.2 g

Cholesterol 13 mg

Sodium 52 mg

Total Carbs 5.5 g

Sugar 1.3 g

Fiber 0.5 g

Protein 6.1 g

Chapter 7. 21-day Meal Plan

DAY	BREAKFAST	MAIN	DESSERT
1)	Best Keto Bread	Gingerbread Spiced Bundt Cake	Chocolate Swirl Buns
2)	Microwave Keto Bread	Cheesy Broccoli Bread	Sesame Buns
3)	Almond Bread	Lemon-Raspberry Quick Bread	Lemon Poppy Seed Muffins
4)	Cinnamon Bread	Pumpkin Quick Bread	Cheesy Herb Muffins
5)	Coconut Bread	Banana-Nut Bread	Chocolate Zucchini Muffins
6)	Sandwich Bread	Cherry, Orange, and Pistachio Quick Bread with Orange Glaze	Pumpkin Spice Muffins
7)	Almond Bread	Lemon–Poppy Seed Bread	Creamy Chocolate Muffins
8)	Multi-Purpose Keto Bread	Skillet Corn Bread	Cinnamon Bagel Bites
9)	Eggy Coconut Bread	Basic Gluten-Free Pie Dough	Almond Flour Bagels
10)	Coconut Flatbread	Sweet Tart Dough	Mozzarella Bagels
11)	Keto Garlic Bread	Double-Crusted Berry Pie	Sour Cream Biscuits

12)	Oopsie Bread Rolls	Key Lime Pie	Hot Dog Buns
13)	Peanut Butter And Chocolate Bread	Pumpkin Pie	Matcha Fudge Bombs
14)	Low Carb Vanilla Bread	Marbled Chocolate and Peanut Butter Pie	Keto Strawberry Fudge
15)	Chocolate Bread	Chocolate Chip Keto Bread	Cream Cheese Delights
16)	Whole Wheat Coconut Bread	Low Carb Bun For One	Pecan Fat Bombs
17)	Garlic, Herb And Cheese Bread	Focaccia Style Flax Bread	Chocolate Fat Bomb
18)	Blackberry Bread	Coconut And Almond Bread	Hamburger Bun
19)	Caprese On Toast	Keto BLT With Oopsie Bread	Spinach Buns
20)	Low Carb Baked Bread	Healthy Cornbread	Angel Food Cake with Coconut Whipped Cream and Strawberries
21)	Keto Blueberry Lemon Bread	Keto Spinach Bread	Cranberry Loaf Cake

Conclusion

Thank you for reading this book and having the patience to try the recipes.

I do hope that you have had as much enjoyment reading and experimenting with the meals as I have had writing the book.